THE
HEALING KITCHEN

Recipes to Soothe Inflammation and Restore Vitality

Robert C. Goff

© 2024 by Robert Goff

All rights reserved. No part of this publication may be reproduced, distributed, or transmitted in any form or by any means, including photocopying, recording, or other electronic or mechanical methods, without the prior written permission of the publisher, except in the case of brief quotations embodied in critical reviews and certain other noncommercial uses permitted by copyright law.

TABLE OF CONTENT

Introduction 5

CHAPTER 1: What is it all about? 6

CHAPTER 2: Why do I need it? 13

CHAPTER 3: How should I go about it? 18

CHAPTER 4: Quick and Easy Breakfasts 43

CHAPTER 5: Snacks and Happy Bites 74

CHAPTER 6: Salads, Wraps and Side Dishes 88

CHAPTER 7: Vegetarian and Vegan 103

CHAPTER 8: Fish and Seafood 117

CHAPTER 9: Poultry and Meats 130

CHAPTER 10: Soups and Stews 148

CHAPTER 11: Condiments, Dressing and Sauces 166

CHAPTER 12: Better Sleep, Minimized Stress Levels and Physical Activity 179

30 Days Meal Plan 185

Recipe Index 193

References 200

Foods Elimination Plan 202

Recipe Journal 214

INTRODUCTION

Hi there! I'm Robert, and I'm very happy that you've chosen to read this book. Prior to delving into the mouthwatering realm of anti-inflammatory cuisine, allow me to briefly discuss the motivation behind writing this book and how it might benefit you.

I was exactly where you were a few years ago. My joints hurt, I was always exhausted, and I felt like my body was rebelling against me. Physicians used terms like "chronic inflammation," but I had no idea how to address it. That's when I came onto the anti-inflammatory food movement, and my life has never been the same!

The truth is, however, that I'm not a health fanatic and I don't think bland, boring cuisine is acceptable. I'm simply an ordinary person who enjoys eating and thinks that eating should be fun. I thus made it my goal to create meals that would both benefit my health and my palate.

You'll learn the outcome of the quest in this book. These aren't simply recipes; I hope you'll use them as your own personal road map to feeling better. I've simplified the science of inflammation into digestible parts so you can understand precisely why you're consuming the foods you are.

Every meal in this book, from filling breakfasts to robust dinners and even some sweets (because life's too short to miss dessert), is created to promote healing in your body and satisfy your palate.

I understand, I promise. Making dietary changes might seem daunting. But I guarantee you, it doesn't have to be. These are easy dishes that won't make you feel deprived since they utilize real, store-bought goods.

I thus cordially encourage you to join me at The Healing Kitchen, whether you are addressing a particular health concern or just want to feel better all around. Together, let's prepare some delectable meals and reduce inflammation.

1: What Is It All About?

Inflammation is a critical aspect of the body's immunological response. It is a complicated biological process that happens when the body senses dangerous stimuli such as germs, damaged cells, or irritants. The basic objective of inflammation is to remove the initial source of cell harm, clear away necrotic cells and tissues damaged by the original insult, and commence tissue healing.

When the body recognizes an injury or illness, it produces an inflammatory reaction. This reaction includes the immune system delivering white blood cells, cytokines, and other inflammatory mediators to the damaged region. These cells and chemicals work together to separate and eliminate the damaging agents and begin the healing process.

Types of Inflammation

- Acute Inflammation: This is a short-term reaction that normally dissipates within a few days. It is characterized by redness, heat, swelling, discomfort, and loss of function. Acute inflammation is useful since it allows the body to swiftly cope with illnesses or injuries.
- Chronic Inflammation: This is a protracted inflammatory reaction that may extend for months or even years. Chronic inflammation may develop from a failure to eradicate the source of acute inflammation, an inflammatory reaction, or continuous exposure to irritants. Unlike acute inflammation, chronic inflammation may lead to tissue damage and contribute to many illnesses such as rheumatoid arthritis, cardiovascular disorders, and certain malignancies.

The Science behind Inflammation

Inflammation is a vital component of the immune system's reaction to damaging stimuli, such as infections, damaged cells, or irritants. When the body senses these dangers, the immune system launches an inflammatory response to protect and repair the afflicted tissues.

The process starts when immune cells, such as macrophages and dendritic cells, identify hazardous chemicals via pattern recognition receptors (PRRs). These receptors detect pathogen-associated molecular patterns (PAMPs) and damage-associated molecular patterns (DAMPs). Upon identification, these cells produce signaling molecules called cytokines, which work as messengers to bring additional immune cells to the site of damage or infection.

The immune system carefully manages inflammation to ensure it is efficient without causing severe harm to the body. Anti-inflammatory cytokines and regulatory T cells (Tregs) serve key roles in suppressing the inflammatory response after the danger is eliminated, limiting persistent inflammation and encouraging tissue healing.

Key Players in Inflammation

Several types of cells and molecules are involved in the inflammatory process:

- Neutrophils: These are the first responders to the site of infection or injury. They engulf and destroy pathogens through a process called phagocytosis.
- Macrophages: These cells also perform phagocytosis and release cytokines to sustain the inflammatory response. They play a role in both initiating and resolving inflammation.
- Lymphocytes: These include T cells and B cells, which are involved in the adaptive immune response. T cells can directly kill infected cells or help other immune cells, while B cells produce antibodies.
- Cytokines: These signaling molecules, such as interleukins, interferons, and tumor necrosis factors, coordinate the immune response by promoting or inhibiting inflammation.
- Chemokines: These are a subset of cytokines that specifically attract immune cells to the site of inflammation.

The Inflammatory Cascade

The inflammatory response can be broken down into several stages:

1. Recognition: Immune cells detect harmful stimuli through PRRs.
2. Activation: The recognition of harmful agents triggers the release of pro-inflammatory cytokines and chemokines.
3. Recruitment: Cytokines and chemokines attract immune cells, such as neutrophils and macrophages, to the site of injury or infection.
4. Elimination: Immune cells work to eliminate the harmful agents through phagocytosis and the release of antimicrobial substances.
5. Resolution: Once the threat is neutralized, anti-inflammatory cytokines and Tregs help to resolve the inflammation and promote tissue repair.

Why Inflammation Matters

When tissues are injured or infected, the body initiates an inflammatory response to contain and eliminate the harmful agents and begin the healing process. This response involves a series of coordinated steps:

1. Vasodilation: Blood vessels in the affected area widen, increasing blood flow. This brings more immune cells, nutrients, and oxygen to the site of injury or infection.
2. Increased Permeability: Blood vessel walls become more permeable, allowing immune cells and proteins to move from the bloodstream into the affected tissues.
3. Migration of Immune Cells: White blood cells, such as neutrophils and macrophages, migrate to the site of injury or infection. These cells engulf and destroy pathogens, remove dead cells, and release signaling molecules to recruit more immune cells.
4. Tissue Repair: Once the harmful agents are neutralized, the body initiates tissue repair. Fibroblasts produce collagen and other extracellular matrix components to rebuild the damaged tissue.

This process is essential for healing wounds, fighting infections, and maintaining overall health.

When It Goes Wrong

While acute inflammation is useful, persistent inflammation may be detrimental. Chronic inflammation occurs when the inflammatory response continues for a long time, resulting in tissue damage and contributing to numerous disorders. Some of the hazards of chronic inflammation include:

- Autoimmune Diseases: Conditions such as rheumatoid arthritis, lupus, and multiple sclerosis occur when the immune system mistakenly attacks the body's own tissues, leading to chronic inflammation and tissue damage.
- Cardiovascular Diseases: Chronic inflammation can contribute to the development of atherosclerosis, where plaques build up in the arteries, increasing the risk of heart attacks and strokes.
- Metabolic Disorders: Chronic inflammation is linked to insulin resistance and type 2 diabetes. Inflammatory cytokines can interfere with insulin signaling, leading to elevated blood sugar levels.
- Cancer: Inflammation can promote the growth and spread of cancer cells by creating an environment that supports tumor development. Chronic inflammation is associated with an increased risk of certain cancers, such as colorectal and liver cancer.

Inflammation in Daily Life

- ❖ After Exercise: Physical activity, particularly vigorous or prolonged exercise, may produce micro-tears in muscle fibers, resulting in inflammation. This is a typical aspect of the muscle regeneration process and helps generate stronger muscles. However, severe inflammation may lead to irritation and harm.
- ❖ Infections: When the body identifies pathogens such as bacteria, viruses, or fungus, it starts an inflammatory response to combat the illness. Symptoms of inflammation, such as fever, redness, and edema, are frequent during infections.
- ❖ Injuries: Cuts, bruises, and other traumas induce inflammation as the body strives to heal damaged tissues. The traditional indications of inflammation—redness, heat, swelling, and pain—are commonly detected near the site of damage.
- ❖ Allergies: Allergic responses occur when the immune system overreacts to innocuous things, such as pollen or pet dander. This stimulates inflammation, resulting in symptoms such as itching, swelling, and redness.

Lifestyle and Environmental Triggers

Inflammation is not only influenced by infections and injuries but also by various lifestyle and environmental factors. These factors can either exacerbate or help manage inflammation, impacting overall health and well-being.

Diet and Inflammation

The foods we eat have a crucial influence in either generating or decreasing inflammation. Certain food choices might provoke inflammatory reactions, while others can help alleviate them.

- Pro-Inflammatory meals: Diets high in refined sugars, trans fats, and processed meals may cause inflammation. These foods may lead to the generation of pro-inflammatory cytokines and contribute to chronic inflammation. Examples include sugary drinks, fried meals, and processed meats.
- Anti-Inflammatory Foods: Conversely, a diet rich in fruits, vegetables, whole grains, and healthy fats may help lower inflammation. Foods strong in omega-3 fatty acids, such as fatty fish, flaxseeds, and walnuts, have anti-inflammatory qualities. Additionally, antioxidants contained in berries, leafy greens, and nuts may help counteract oxidative stress and inflammation.

Stress and Inflammation

Chronic stress is a well-known cause for inflammation. When the body is under stress, it releases stress hormones like cortisol and adrenaline. While these hormones are needed for the "fight or flight" response, chronic stress may lead to an imbalance, resulting in increased production of pro-inflammatory cytokines.

- Psychological Stress: Mental health disorders such as anxiety and depression are connected to greater levels of inflammation. Chronic stress may impair the immune system, making the body more prone to infections and inflammatory illnesses.
- Physical Stress: Overtraining or excessive physical activity without appropriate rest may also cause inflammation. While moderate exercise is helpful, pushing the body beyond its limitations may cause muscular injury and inflammation.

Pollution and Inflammation

Environmental contaminants, including air pollution, chemicals, and poisons, may substantially contribute to inflammation. Exposure to contaminants may activate an immunological response, leading to persistent inflammation and different health concerns.

- Air Pollution: Particulate matter, ozone, and other pollutants in the air may induce respiratory inflammation and worsen illnesses including asthma and chronic obstructive pulmonary disease (COPD). Long-term exposure to air pollution is also connected to cardiovascular illnesses and systemic inflammation.
- Chemical Exposure: Pesticides, industrial chemicals, and home cleansers may include compounds that provoke inflammatory reactions. These substances may affect the endocrine system and lead to chronic inflammation and illnesses such as cancer and autoimmune disorders.

Other Factors Influencing Inflammation

Several other lifestyle and environmental factors can impact inflammation:

- Sleep: Poor sleep quality and inadequate sleep might promote inflammation. Sleep is necessary for the body's healing processes, and persistent sleep loss may lead to high levels of inflammatory markers.
- Obesity: Excess body fat, especially visceral fat, may create proinflammatory cytokines. Obesity is connected with persistent low-grade inflammation, which may lead to metabolic problems, cardiovascular illnesses, and other health difficulties.
- Smoking: Tobacco smoke includes several chemicals that may cause inflammation in the lungs and other organs of the body. Smoking is a substantial risk factor for chronic inflammatory illnesses such as COPD and cardiovascular disorders.
- Alcohol: Excessive alcohol use may lead to liver inflammation and damage. Chronic alcohol usage is related with an increased risk of inflammatory diseases such as alcoholic hepatitis and pancreatitis.

Managing Inflammation through Lifestyle Changes

- Balanced Diet: Focus on a diet rich in anti-inflammatory foods, such as fruits, vegetables, whole grains, and healthy fats. Limit the consumption of processed foods, refined carbohydrates, and trans fats.
- Stress Management: Practice stress-reducing strategies such as mindfulness, meditation, yoga, and deep breathing exercises. Regular physical exercise and hobbies may also help ease stress.
- Adequate Sleep: Aim for 7-9 hours of decent sleep each night. Establish a consistent sleep schedule and establish a comfortable sleep environment.
- Avoiding Pollutants: Reduce exposure to environmental pollutants by utilizing natural cleaning products, avoiding smoking, and reducing time spent in extremely polluted locations.
- Regular Exercise: Engage in regular physical exercise, but avoid overtraining. Moderate exercise may help decrease inflammation and enhance overall health.

2: Why Do I Need it?

The Gut-Inflammation Connection

The health of our gut plays a critical role in managing inflammation throughout the body. The gut is home to billions of bacteria, collectively known as the gut microbiome, which have a substantial influence on our immune system and inflammatory reactions.

The gut microbiome consists of a varied collection of bacteria, viruses, fungus, and other microbes. A healthy gut microbiota helps preserve the integrity of the gut lining, aids digestion, and controls the immune system. However, an imbalance in the gut microbiota, known as dysbiosis, may contribute to increased inflammation.

Factors Influencing Gut Health

Several variables may alter the health of the gut microbiome and, subsequently, inflammation:

- Diet: A diet strong in fiber, fruits, vegetables, and fermented foods promotes a healthy gut flora. Conversely, diets high in processed foods, sweets, and bad fats may disturb the equilibrium of gut microbes.
- Antibiotics: While antibiotics are crucial for treating bacterial infections, they may also disturb the gut microbiota by killing beneficial bacteria. This disturbance may lead to increased inflammation.
- Stress: Chronic stress may adversely affect gut health by changing the makeup of the gut microbiota and increasing intestinal permeability, which can promote inflammation.

Gut-Brain Axis

The stomach and brain are linked via a complex network known as the gut-brain axis. This bidirectional communication system incorporates the neurological system, hormones, and immunological signals. The gut microbiota may impact brain function and mood, and vice versa, underscoring the relevance of gut health in general well-being.

Managing Inflammation through Diet

To control and minimize inflammation, it is necessary to concentrate on a diet that promotes gut health and contains anti-inflammatory foods. Here are some dietary strategies:

- Increase Fiber Intake: Consuming a range of fiber-rich foods, such as fruits, vegetables, legumes, and whole grains, maintains a healthy gut flora and decreases inflammation
- Include Fermented Foods: Foods like yogurt, kefir, sauerkraut, and kimchi include probiotics that support a healthy balance of intestinal flora.
- Limit Processed Foods: Reducing the consumption of processed and sugary meals may help avoid dysbiosis and decrease inflammation
- Stay Hydrated: Drinking enough of water improves digestion and helps maintain a healthy gut lining.

Common inflammatory conditions and symptoms

1. Rheumatoid Arthritis (RA)

An autoimmune condition called rheumatoid arthritis occurs when the immune system unintentionally targets the joints, leading to inflammation.

Symptoms:
- Joint pain and stiffness, especially in the morning or after periods of inactivity.
- Swelling and tenderness in the joints.
- Fatigue and general malaise.
- Fever and weight loss in severe cases

2. Inflammatory Bowel Disease (IBD)

IBD includes diseases that cause persistent inflammation of the gastrointestinal system, such as ulcerative colitis and Crohn's disease.

Symptoms:
- Abdominal pain and cramping.
- Diarrhea, often with blood or mucus.
- Weight loss and malnutrition.
- Fatigue and fever.

3. Psoriasis

Psoriasis is a chronic skin condition characterized by an overactive immune response that leads to the rapid buildup of skin cells.

Symptoms:
- Red, scaly patches of skin, often covered with silvery scales.
- Itching and burning sensations.
- Dry, cracked skin that may bleed.
- Swollen and stiff joints in psoriatic arthritis[3].

4. Asthma

Asthma is a chronic respiratory condition where inflammation and narrowing of the airways cause difficulty in breathing.

Symptoms:
- Shortness of breath and wheezing.
- Chest tightness.
- Coughing, especially at night or early morning.
- Increased mucus production[4].

5. Lupus

Lupus is an autoimmune disease that can affect various parts of the body, including the skin, joints, kidneys, and brain.

Symptoms:

- Fatigue and fever.
- Joint pain, stiffness, and swelling.
- Skin rashes, often in a butterfly shape across the cheeks and nose.
- Sensitivity to sunlight.
- Kidney problems and chest pain.

6. Chronic Obstructive Pulmonary Disease (COPD)

COPD is a group of lung diseases, including emphysema and chronic bronchitis, characterized by chronic inflammation of the airways.

Symptoms:
- Persistent cough with mucus production.
- Shortness of breath, especially during physical activities.
- Frequent respiratory infections.
- Wheezing and chest tightness.

7. Multiple Sclerosis (MS)

MS is an autoimmune disease where the immune system attacks the protective covering of nerves, leading to inflammation and damage.

Symptoms:
- Numbness or weakness in limbs.
- Loss of vision, often in one eye at a time.
- Tingling or pain in parts of the body.
- Tremors and lack of coordination.

8. Type 1 Diabetes

Type 1 diabetes is an autoimmune condition where the immune system attacks insulin-producing cells in the pancreas, leading to inflammation.

Symptoms:
- Increased thirst and frequent urination.
- Extreme hunger and unintended weight loss.
- Fatigue and weakness.

- Blurred vision.

9. Chronic Sinusitis

Chronic sinusitis is a condition where the sinuses become inflamed and swollen for an extended period, often due to infection or allergies.

Symptoms:
- Nasal congestion and discharge.
- Pain and tenderness around the eyes, cheeks, nose, and forehead.
- Reduced sense of smell and taste.
- Cough and sore throat.

10. Ankylosing Spondylitis

Ankylosing spondylitis is a type of arthritis that primarily affects the spine, causing inflammation and leading to chronic pain and stiffness.

Symptoms:
- Lower back pain and stiffness, especially in the morning or after periods of inactivity.
- Pain and swelling in other joints, such as the hips and shoulders.
- Fatigue and reduced flexibility.
- In severe cases, the spine may become fused.

3: How Should I Go About It?

Leafy greens are nutritional powerhouses that provide a broad variety of health advantages, especially when it comes to reducing inflammation in the body. Incorporating leafy greens into your diet may help counteract this inflammation and boost overall health.

One of the primary reasons leafy greens are so helpful at decreasing inflammation is their high amount of antioxidants. These substances help neutralize free radicals in the body, which may cause cellular damage and lead to inflammation. Leafy greens are especially rich in vitamins C and E, beta-carotene, and flavonoids, all of which have significant antioxidant qualities.

Additionally, many leafy greens include omega-3 fatty acids, which are recognized for their anti-inflammatory benefits. While not as concentrated as in fatty fish, the omega-3s in leafy greens may nevertheless contribute to an overall anti-inflammatory diet.

Leafy greens are also good providers of dietary nitrates, which the body converts to nitric oxide. Nitric oxide helps dilate blood vessels, boosting blood flow and perhaps lowering inflammation throughout the body.

Some of the greatest leafy greens for combating inflammation include:

1. Spinach: Rich in antioxidants and anti-inflammatory substances including quercetin and kaempferol.
2. Kale: Packed in vitamins A, C, and K, as well as antioxidants like quercetin and kaempferol.
3. Collard greens: High in vitamins A, C, and K, and include glucosinolates that may help decrease inflammation.
4. Swiss chard: Contains betalains, antioxidants with anti-inflammatory qualities.

5. Arugula: Rich in glucosinolates and other substances that may help decrease inflammation.

Nutritional Benefits of Leafy Greens

Beyond their anti-inflammatory qualities, leafy greens provide a broad variety of nutritional benefits:

- Low in calories: Leafy greens are very nutrient-dense while being low in calories, making them good for weight control.
- High in fiber: The fiber in leafy greens improves digestive health, helps maintain blood sugar levels, and increases feelings of fullness.
- Rich in vitamins and minerals: Leafy greens are good providers of vitamins A, C, E, and K, as well as folate, iron, magnesium, potassium, and calcium.
- Phytonutrients: These plants include numerous beneficial chemicals including lutein and zeaxanthin, which improve eye health.
- Hydration: Many leafy greens contain significant water content, adding to general hydration.
- Alkalizing effect: Leafy greens may help regulate the body's pH levels, thereby lowering the risk of chronic illnesses.

How to Choose the Best Leafy Greens

To obtain the most nutritional value from your leafy greens, it's crucial to pick the freshest and highest-quality alternatives available. Here are some tips:

1. Look for lively colors: The leaves should be rich green without any fading or browning.
2. Check for crispness: Leaves should be crisp and firm, not wilted or greasy.
3. Avoid damaged leaves: Steer clear of greens with holes, rips, or evidence of insect damage.
4. Consider organic options: While not always essential, organic greens may contain reduced pesticide residues.
5. Buy in season: Seasonal greens are frequently fresher and more nutrient-dense.
6. Check the stems: For greens like kale or, chard, ensure the stems are sturdy and not too woody.

7. Smell test: Fresh leafy greens should have a clear, fresh aroma without any off scents.
8. Consider pre-washed options: If convenience is a necessity, pre-washed greens might be a fine choice, but always rinse them before use.

How I Prepare Leafy Greens

I've developed a few go-to techniques for cooking leafy greens since I adore them in my diet. This is my own methodology:

I always give leafy greens a good wash as soon as I get them home from the market. I prefer to rinse them under cold running water to get rid of any last bits of dirt or debris, even if they've already been cleaned. To make sure heartier greens like kale are clean, I'll soak them for approximately five minutes in a basin of cold water with a dash of vinegar.

I dry the greens with a salad spinner after washing. This is an important step since too much water may dilute salad dressings and make cooked greens mushy. I'll use paper towels or a fresh kitchen towel to gently pat the greens dry if I don't have a salad spinner.

I often massage harder greens, like kale, for raw recipes. I'll sprinkle the leaves with a little olive oil and salt, then give them a minute or two of gentle massage with my hands. As a result, the kale becomes more soft and simpler to digest as the fibers are broken down.

In terms of cooking, I have a few go-to techniques. I frequently sauté my greens for a simple and fast meal. I add some minced garlic to a skillet with a little olive or coconut oil, heat it up, and then add the greens. Typically, a fast stir-fry of three to five minutes is sufficient to wilt the greens without sacrificing their rich color and nutrients.

I could cook collards or other heartier greens for a longer time. I'll trim off any stiff stems before slicing the leaves into tiny strips. After that, I'll cook them in a saucepan with some garlic, chopped onion, and stock. Towards the conclusion of the cooking process, add a splash of apple cider vinegar to help tenderize the greens and offer a wonderful tangy taste.

To add extra nutrients to smoothies, I also like using leafy greens. I usually use spinach for this since it goes well with fruits because of its mild taste. For a quick and nutritious breakfast, I'll throw some frozen fruit, Greek yogurt, and a splash of almond milk into a blender with a handful of fresh spinach.

Finally, I make it a point to have raw leafy greens in all of my meals. Adding additional greens to my diet is as easy as making a simple side salad with mixed greens and homemade vinaigrette. For an added crunch and good fats, I usually sprinkle some nuts or seeds on top of the salad.

I make sure I'm receiving a variety of nutrients from my leafy greens and never grow tired of my meals by cooking them in different ways. These adaptable veggies, whether they are cooked or raw, are a mainstay of my diet.

Anti-Inflammatory Benefits of Omega-3 Fatty Acids

One important function of omega-3 fatty acids, a kind of polyunsaturated fats, is to lower inflammation throughout the body. There are three primary varieties of omega-3s:

1. Eicosapentaenoic acid, or EPA
2. Docosahexaenoic acid, or DHA
3. Alpha-linolenic acid, or ALA

Walnuts, chia seeds, and flaxseeds are plant sources of ALA, whereas fatty fish and fish oil are the main sources of EPA, DHA, and ALA.

It is well known that omega-3 fatty acids, particularly EPA and DHA, have anti-inflammatory properties. These fats have several anti-inflammatory effects:

1. Limiting the production of pro-inflammatory cytokines: Omega-3 fatty acids have the ability to reduce the synthesis of pro-inflammatory cytokines such as tumor necrosis factor (TNF), interleukin-1 (IL-1), and interleukin-6 (IL-6).
2. Generating anti-inflammatory substances: When omega-3s are ingested, they are transformed into substances known as proteins and resolvins, which actively assist in reducing inflammation in the body.

3. Maintaining a balanced omega-6 to omega-3 ratio: The majority of Western diets include a lot of omega-6 fatty acids, which, when taken in excess, may exacerbate inflammation. Ingesting more omega-3s contributes to balancing this imbalance and lowering general inflammation.
4. Inhibiting inflammatory enzymes: Cyclooxygenase-2 (COX-2) and other enzymes implicated in inflammatory processes may have their activity decreased by omega-3 fatty acids.
5. Modifying the composition of cell membranes: Omega-3s may modify the way cells react to inflammatory signals by integrating into their membranes.

Advantages of Omega-3 Fatty Acids for Health

Numerous health advantages are facilitated by omega-3 fatty acids' anti-inflammatory properties, including:

1. Cardiovascular Health: Omega-3 fatty acids mitigate the risk of heart attack and stroke, lower blood pressure, lessen blood clotting, and lessen irregular heartbeats.
2. Mental Health and Brain Function: DHA is an important structural element of the brain. Sufficient consumption of omega-3 fatty acids is linked to a lower risk of Alzheimer's disease and cognitive decline, and it may also aid in the treatment of anxiety and depression.
3. Eye Health: A significant structural element of the retina is DHA. Omega-3 fatty acids may be able to stop dry eye condition and macular degeneration.
4. Pregnancy and Early Life: The development of the fetal brain and eyes depends on an adequate omega-3 diet throughout pregnancy. Also, it could lessen the chance of premature delivery.
5. Autoimmune Diseases: Psoriasis, lupus, rheumatoid arthritis, ulcerative colitis, and Crohn's disease are a few autoimmune diseases that omega-3 fatty acids may help treat.
6. Cancer Prevention: Research indicates that omega-3 fatty acids may help lower the incidence of some malignancies, including prostate, breast, and colon cancer.
7. Bone and Joint Health: Omega-3 fatty acids may help lower bone loss, enhance calcium absorption, and alleviate rheumatoid arthritis symptoms.
8. Skin Health: Omega-3 fatty acids are critical for maintaining healthy skin and may aid in the treatment of dermatitis and psoriasis.

9. Weight Management: Omega-3s may assist lower fat accumulation and increase insulin sensitivity, but they are not a magic bullet for weight reduction.
10. Liver Health: For those with non-alcoholic fatty liver disease, omega-3 fatty acids may help lower liver fat.

How I Use Omega-3 Fatty Acids

I'm very interested in nutrition and health, therefore I've tried to include omega-3 fatty acids in my daily routine as much as possible. I make sure I receive enough of these healthy fats in the following ways:

Dietary Sources:

I make an effort to eat fatty fish twice a week or more. Sardines, mackerel, and salmon are always my first picks. I really like to make a fast sardine salad for lunch or grill salmon with some herbs and a splash of lemon. I sometimes eat canned tuna when I'm pressed for time, but I try not to eat it too often because of mercury concerns.

I often incorporate ground flaxseed and chia seeds in my diet for plant-based omega-3s. I often use them to smoothies or sprinkle them over my yogurt or cereal in the morning. Another common item in my cupboard is walnuts; I like to add them to salads for crunch or just nibble on a tiny bunch as a snack.

Additionally, because canola or flaxseed oils are excellent sources of ALA, I make an effort to utilize them in my cooking whenever possible.

Supplements:

To make sure I'm receiving enough omega-3s from whole foods, I now take a premium fish oil supplement in addition to putting real foods first. I looked for a supplement that has undergone independent testing to ensure its efficacy and integrity. In order to enhance absorption, I take it after a meal that includes some fat.

I avoid taking too much of my supplement on days when I eat fish. It's also important to note that I spoke with my doctor before beginning any supplement regimen.

Omega-6 to Omega-3 Ratio Balancing: In order to get a better balance, I'm aware that I should be consuming less omega-6 and more omega-3. This means that I try to cook with olive oil rather than vegetable oils high in omega-6 fatty acids and have reduced my intake of processed meals.

Tracking Intake:

I regularly keep an eye on my omega-3 consumption using a nutrition monitoring app. This helps me make sure I always receive enough, particularly during the periods when I may not have had as much fish as normal.

Cooking Methods:

I take care not to overcook meals high in omega-3s since excessive heat may destroy these sensitive lipids. For fish, I often use lower-heat cooking techniques like poaching or gentle sautéing. To avoid oxidation, I also keep my omega-3-rich oils in a cold, dark spot.

Combining with Other Nutrients:

I now know that eating some additional nutrients alongside omega-3s may improve their absorption. For example, I often combine meals high in omega-3 with fat-soluble vitamins, such as vitamin D (which I receive via sunshine exposure and fortified foods) and vitamin E (found in nuts and seeds).

Fermented Foods and Gut Health

Since ancient times, humans have used fermented foods in their diets because of their distinct tastes, capacity for preservation, and several health advantages. These foods have seen a rise in popularity recently, especially because of their beneficial impact on gut health.

Foods that have gone through the lacto fermentation process, in which natural bacteria consume the food's sugar and starch to produce lactic acid, are referred to as fermented foods. In addition to producing healthy enzymes, B vitamins, omega-3 fatty acids, and different probiotic strains, this procedure protects the food.

Common examples of fermented foods include:

1. Yogurt
2. Kefir
3. Sauerkraut
4. Kimchi
5. Kombucha
6. Miso
7. Tempeh
8. Pickles (fermented, not vinegar-based)
9. Natto
10. Sourdough bread

Benefits of Fermented Foods for Gut Health

1. Introducing Beneficial Bacteria

The probiotic content of fermented foods is the main advantage for gut health. Probiotics are living bacteria that provide the host health benefits when taken in sufficient quantities. These good bacteria may aid in the colonization of the stomach with germs that support health.

Different probiotic strains may be found in different fermented foods. As an illustration: Lactobacillus bulgaricus and Streptococcus thermophilus are often found in yogurt.
- Kefir might include as many as 61 distinct microbes in it.
- Lactobacillus plantarum, L. brevis, and L. acidophilus are abundant in sauerkraut.

Maintaining a healthy gut flora is essential for general health, and these probiotics may assist.

2. Improving Digestive Function

Fermented foods can aid digestion in several ways:

- Enzyme production: The fermentation process creates enzymes that can help break down food, making nutrients more easily absorbable.

- Reducing lactose: For dairy products, fermentation can break down lactose, making these foods more tolerable for people with lactose intolerance.
- Fiber content: Many fermented plant-based foods are high in fiber, which aids digestion and promotes regular bowel movements.

3. Enhancing Nutrient Absorption

The process of fermentation can increase the bioavailability of nutrients in food. For example:
- Fermentation can increase the availability of vitamins, particularly B vitamins.
- It can enhance mineral absorption by reducing phytic acid, which can interfere with mineral absorption.

4. Supporting the Immune System

About 70% of our immune system is located in the gut. By promoting a healthy gut microbiome, fermented foods can indirectly support immune function. Some studies suggest that certain probiotic strains can stimulate the production of natural antibodies in the body.

5. Reducing Inflammation

Chronic inflammation in the gut can lead to various health issues. Some studies suggest that certain probiotic strains found in fermented foods may help reduce inflammation in the gut, potentially alleviating symptoms of inflammatory bowel diseases like ulcerative colitis.

6. Improving Symptoms of Irritable Bowel Syndrome (IBS)

Some research indicates that certain probiotics found in fermented foods may help alleviate symptoms of IBS, such as bloating, gas, and irregular bowel movements.

7. Potential Mental Health Benefits

There's a growing body of research exploring the gut-brain axis, suggesting that gut health can influence mental health. Some studies have found associations between probiotic consumption and reduced symptoms of anxiety and depression.

8. Producing Short-Chain Fatty Acids

When probiotics ferment fiber in the colon, they produce short-chain fatty acids (SCFAs). These compounds play several important roles in gut health, including:
- Providing energy for colon cells
- Reducing inflammation
- Improving mineral absorption
- Potentially reducing the risk of colorectal cancer

9. Supporting Weight Management

While more research is needed, some studies suggest that certain probiotic strains may help with weight management by influencing appetite-regulating hormones and fat storage.

10. Reducing Antibiotic-Associated Diarrhea

Probiotics found in fermented foods may help prevent or reduce diarrhea associated with antibiotic use by repopulating the gut with beneficial bacteria.

Incorporating Fermented Foods into Your Diet

To reap the gut health benefits of fermented foods, it's important to incorporate them regularly into your diet. Here are some tips:

1. Start small: If you're new to fermented foods, start with small amounts and gradually increase to avoid potential digestive discomfort.

2. Diversity is key: Try to include a variety of fermented foods to expose your gut to different probiotic strains.

3. Look for "live and active cultures": When buying yogurt or other fermented products, look for this phrase on the label to ensure you're getting live probiotics.

4. Consider homemade options: Making your own fermented foods like sauerkraut or kefir can be a fun and cost-effective way to ensure you're getting high-quality, probiotic-rich foods.

5. Pair with prebiotics: Consuming prebiotic foods (like garlic, onions, and bananas) alongside fermented foods can help feed the beneficial bacteria.

Considerations and Precautions

While fermented foods offer numerous benefits, it's important to keep a few things in mind:

- Some people may experience bloating or gas when first introducing fermented foods. Start with small amounts and increase gradually.
- Individuals with compromised immune systems should consult a healthcare provider before significantly increasing their intake of fermented foods.
- Some fermented foods are high in sodium or calories, so be mindful of portion sizes.
- If you have histamine sensitivity, be aware that some fermented foods are high in histamines.

Olive Oil Kitchen Transformation

For millennia, olive oil, sometimes known as "liquid gold," has been a mainstay in Mediterranean cuisine. Because of its full taste, adaptability, and health advantages, it's a great option to upgrade your cooking and improve your culinary adventures.

Prior to exploring its transforming potential, it's essential to comprehend what makes olive oil unique:

1. Production: Olive oil is derived from the fruit of olive trees. Extra virgin olive oil (EVOO) is the finest quality, derived from the initial cold pressing of olives without using heat or chemicals.
2. Grades: Olive oil comes in numerous grades, including extra virgin, virgin, and refined. EVOO is the most coveted for its taste and health advantages.

3. Flavor profiles: Olive oils may vary from light and buttery to powerful and peppery, depending on variables including olive type, maturity, and manufacturing processes.

Cooking with Olive Oil

One of the most important ways olive oil can improve your kitchen is by becoming your go-to cooking oil. Here's how:

1. Sautéing and Stir-frying: Use olive oil instead of butter or vegetable oils for a healthier option that gives a mild, fruity taste to your recipes.
2. Roasting: Toss vegetables or meats in olive oil before roasting to improve taste and encourage crispy exteriors.
3. Grilling: Brush olive oil on items before grilling to avoid sticking and enhance taste.
4. Baking: Substitute olive oil for other fats in baking recipes for moist, tasty results.
5. Pasta dishes: Finish pasta meals with a drizzle of high-quality EVOO for extra depth and richness.
6. Marinades: Create delectable marinades using olive oil as a foundation, mixed with herbs, spices, and acidity like lemon juice or vinegar.
7. Dressings: Make homemade salad dressings with olive oil for fresher, healthier alternatives to store-bought ones.

Flavor Enhancement

Olive oil may modify the taste character of your dishes:

- Infusions: Create herb or spice-infused olive oils for distinctive flavor accents to your cuisine.
- Finishing oil: Use a high-quality EVOO as a finishing oil over soups, stews, or grilled meats to give a layer of taste and richness.
- Dipping: Serve crusty bread with olive oil for dipping, maybe with additional herbs or balsamic vinegar.
- Emulsions: Use olive oil to produce stable emulsions for sauces like mayonnaise or aioli.

Health Benefits

Transforming your kitchen with olive oil isn't only about flavor—it's also about health:

1. Heart health: The monounsaturated fats in olive oil may help decrease harmful cholesterol levels and lessen the risk of heart disease.

2. Anti-inflammatory properties: Olive oil includes oleocanthal, a molecule having anti-inflammatory actions comparable to ibuprofen.

3. Antioxidants: Rich in vitamin E and other antioxidants, olive oil may help counteract oxidative stress in the body.

4. Brain health: Some research shows that a Mediterranean diet rich in olive oil may help prevent cognitive decline and lessen the risk of Alzheimer's disease.

5. Digestive health: Olive oil may assist promote digestion and may have good benefits on gut flora.

Kitchen Organization and Storage

Incorporating olive oil into your kitchen extends beyond cooking:

- Olive oil station: Create a designated place for your olive oils, potentially with a range of sorts for various needs.
- Proper storage: Store olive oil in a cold, dark area to retain its quality. Consider using dark glass bottles or tins to shield it from light.
- Olive oil dispenser: Invest in an excellent quality dispenser for simple pouring and appealing display.
- Labeling: If you have various varieties of olive oil, mark them properly with their grade and any taste comments.

Sustainable Kitchen Practices

Olive oil may help to a more sustainable kitchen:

- Reusable containers: Use olive oil spray bottles instead of aerosol cans for a more eco-friendly choice.

- Local sourcing: Look for locally produced olive oils to support local agriculture and decrease transportation-related carbon emissions
- Multi-use product: Use olive oil as a natural furniture polish or to condition wooden cutting boards, minimizing the need for specialist goods.

Culinary Exploration

1. Mediterranean cuisine: Explore classic Mediterranean dishes that extensively incorporate olive oil.

2. Olive oil tastings: Organize olive oil tastings to educate yourself and others about various kinds and taste characteristics.

3. Olive oil pairings: Learn to combine different olive oils with diverse dishes, much like wine pairings.

4. Cooking methods: Master techniques like confit, where meals are slow-cooked in olive oil at low temperatures.

Economic Considerations

While high-quality olive oil might be more costly than some other cooking oils, consider:

- Health advantages: The possible long-term health benefits may justify the greater upfront expense.
- Flavor impact: A little goes a long way in terms of flavor, possibly eliminating the need for additional pricey components.
- Versatility: The multi-use nature of olive oil may replace various other goods in your kitchen.

Challenges and Solutions

Transforming your cooking with olive oil may come with some challenges:

- Smoke point concerns: While EVOO has a greater smoke point than popularly assumed, use lighter olive oils for high-heat cooking if worried.

- Flavor adjustments: Some recipes may require altering when replacing olive oil with other fats. Experiment and modify to your taste.
- Quality assurance: Learn to recognize high-quality olive oils and be aware of mislabeled or contaminated goods.

Anti-Inflammatory Spices: Nature's Powerful Healers

1. Turmeric

Turmeric is perhaps the most well-known anti-inflammatory spice, thanks to its active compound, curcumin.

Benefits:
- Potent anti-inflammatory and antioxidant properties
- May help in managing arthritis symptoms
- Potential to improve brain function and lower risk of brain diseases
- May lower risk of heart disease
- Possible anti-cancer properties

How to use:
- Add to curries, soups, and rice dishes
- Make golden milk by mixing with warm plant-based milk and honey
- Blend into smoothies
- Use in salad dressings

Pro tip: Combine with black pepper to enhance curcumin absorption.

2. Ginger

Ginger has been used for centuries in various traditional medicine systems.

Benefits:
- Reduces inflammation, particularly in the gastrointestinal tract
- May help relieve nausea and motion sickness
- Potential to reduce muscle pain and soreness

- May lower blood sugar levels and improve heart disease risk factors

How to use:
- Brew fresh ginger tea
- Add to stir-fries and marinades
- Use in baked goods like gingerbread
- Blend into smoothies or juices

3. Cinnamon

This sweet spice is not only delicious but also packed with health benefits.

Benefits:
- Contains powerful antioxidants
- May help lower blood sugar levels and improve insulin sensitivity
- Potential to reduce risk factors for heart disease
- May have beneficial effects on neurodegenerative diseases

How to use:
- Sprinkle on oatmeal or yogurt
- Add to baked goods
- Use in savory dishes like Moroccan tagines
- Brew cinnamon tea

4. Garlic

While often considered an herb, garlic's potent medicinal properties earn it a place on this list.

Benefits:
- Contains allicin, a compound with strong anti-inflammatory properties
- May help lower blood pressure and cholesterol levels
- Potential to boost immune function
- Possible anti-cancer properties

How to use:
- Add to savory dishes of all kinds

- Roast whole garlic bulbs for a milder, sweeter flavor
- Use raw in dressings and dips (for maximum health benefits)

5. Cayenne Pepper

This spicy pepper contains capsaicin, which gives it both its heat and many of its health benefits.

Benefits:
- May help reduce pain and inflammation
- Potential to boost metabolism and aid in weight management
- May improve digestive health
- Possible cardiovascular benefits

How to use:
- Add to soups, stews, and chili
- Use in spice rubs for meats
- Sprinkle on roasted vegetables
- Add a pinch to hot chocolate for a spicy twist

6. Cloves

These aromatic flower buds are rich in antioxidants and anti-inflammatory compounds.

Benefits:
- Contains eugenol, a potent anti-inflammatory compound
- May help protect against cancer
- Potential to improve liver health
- May help regulate blood sugar

How to use:
- Use in baked goods and desserts
- Add to mulled wine or cider
- Use in savory meat dishes
- Brew clove tea

7. Rosemary

This fragrant herb is not only delicious but also offers numerous health benefits.

Benefits:
- Contains rosmarinic acid and carnosic acid, which have strong anti-inflammatory and antioxidant properties
- May improve digestion and boost the immune system
- Potential to improve brain function and memory
- May help reduce allergic reactions and nasal congestion

How to use:
- Use to season roasted meats and vegetables
- Add to homemade bread or focaccia
- Infuse in olive oil for a flavorful cooking oil
- Brew rosemary tea

8. Black Pepper

Often overlooked, black pepper contains piperine, a compound with significant health benefits.

Benefits:
- Anti-inflammatory and antioxidant properties
- Enhances the absorption of other nutrients, particularly curcumin from turmeric
- May improve digestion
- Potential to enhance brain function

How to use:
- Grind fresh over almost any savory dish
- Use in spice rubs and marinades
- Add to salad dressings
- Combine with turmeric for enhanced benefits

Adopting Anti-Inflammatory Spices in Your Diet

1. Start Gradually: If you're not accustomed to eating spicy meals, start with tiny portions and gradually increase.

2. Experiment with Combinations: Many of these spices work nicely together. Try various combinations to discover your favorite tastes.
3. Use in Various Forms: Many spices may be used fresh, dried, or as supplements. However, always talk with a healthcare physician before beginning any supplement program.
4. Consider Quality: Opt for high-quality, organic spices wherever feasible to provide optimum benefits and taste.
5. Store Properly: Keep spices in sealed containers away from heat and light to retain their strength.
6. Be Consistent: Regular use is crucial to obtaining the anti-inflammatory effects of these spices.
7. Balance with Other Healthy Habits: While these spices are useful, they operate best as part of an overall healthy diet and lifestyle.

Potential Precautions

While these spices are typically safe for most individuals, it's crucial to note:

- Some spices may interfere with certain drugs. For example, turmeric may interact with blood thinners
- Excessive use of certain spices, like cinnamon, may have detrimental consequences.
- If you have any current health concerns or are pregnant, contact a healthcare practitioner before drastically increasing your consumption of these spices.

Safe to eat Foods

Fruits
- Berries: Blueberries, strawberries, raspberries, blackberries
- Citrus: Oranges, lemons, limes, grapefruits
- Tropical Fruits: Pineapple, mango, papaya
- Stone Fruits: Cherries, plums, peaches
- Apples
- Pears
- Pomegranates

- Grapes

Vegetables
- Leafy Greens: Spinach, kale, Swiss chard, collard greens
- Cruciferous Vegetables: Broccoli, cauliflower, Brussels sprouts, cabbage
- Root Vegetables: Sweet potatoes, carrots, beets, parsnips
- Alliums: Garlic, onions, leeks, shallots
- Peppers: Bell peppers, chili peppers
- Tomatoes
- Zucchini
- Squash: Butternut, acorn, spaghetti squash

Whole Grains
- Quinoa
- Brown Rice
- Oats
- Buckwheat
- Barley
- Millet
- Teff
- Amaranth

Legumes
- Lentils
- Chickpeas
- Black Beans
- Kidney Beans
- Peas
- Navy Beans
- Adzuki Beans

Nuts and Seeds
- Almonds
- Walnuts
- Chia Seeds

- Flaxseeds
- Pumpkin Seeds
- Sunflower Seeds
- Hemp Seeds
- Pine Nuts

Healthy Fats and Oils
- Extra Virgin Olive Oil
- Avocado Oil
- Coconut Oil
- Flaxseed Oil
- Walnut Oil
- Hemp Seed Oil
- Chia Seed Oil
- Macadamia Nut Oil
- Almond Oil

Herbs and Spices
- Turmeric
- Ginger
- Garlic
- Cinnamon
- Cloves
- Rosemary
- Thyme
- Basil
- Oregano
- Cayenne Pepper
- Black Pepper

Fish and Seafood
- Fatty Fish: Salmon, mackerel, sardines, trout, herring
- Shellfish: Shrimp, crab, lobster

- Oysters
- Tuna (especially wild-caught)

Fermented Foods
- Kefir (can be dairy or coconut-based)
- Sauerkraut
- Kimchi
- Tempeh
- Miso
- Kombucha
- Pickles (naturally fermented)

Beverages
- Green Tea
- Herbal Teas: Chamomile, ginger, turmeric tea
- Water with Lemon
- Turmeric Latte
- Bone Broth

Anti-Inflammatory Sweeteners
- Honey (in moderation)
- Maple Syrup (in moderation)
- Molasses (in moderation)
- Stevia (natural, not the highly processed form)

Other Anti-Inflammatory Foods
- Dark Chocolate (70% cocoa or higher)
- Apple Cider Vinegar
- Coconut Milk
- Almond Milk (unsweetened)
- Nutritional Yeast

Foods and Oil to Avoid

Refined and Processed Oils
- Vegetable Oils: Corn oil, soybean oil, sunflower oil (high in omega-6 fatty acids, which can promote inflammation when consumed in excess
- Canola Oil (often highly processed and may contain trans fats)
- Margarine and Shortening (contains trans fats)
- Hydrogenated Oils (often found in processed foods)

Sugary Foods and Beverages
- Refined Sugars: White sugar, high-fructose corn syrup
- Sugary Beverages: Sodas, energy drinks, sweetened teas
- Candy and Sweets
- Pastries and Baked Goods (especially those made with refined flour and sugar)
- Sugary Breakfast Cereals

Refined Carbohydrates
- White Bread
- White Pasta
- White Rice
- Pastries
- Crackers
- Processed Snack Foods: Chips, pretzels

Processed Meats
- Sausages
- Hot Dogs
- Bacon
- Deli Meats
- Salami
- Pepperoni

Fried Foods
- French Fries
- Fried Chicken
- Doughnuts

- Fried Snacks (like potato chips)

Red and Processed Meats
- Beef, Pork, and Lamb (especially when not grass-fed)
- Processed Meats: Bacon, hot dogs, sausages, and deli meats (high in sodium and preservatives)

Dairy Products (for some people)
- Whole Milk
- Cheese (especially processed cheeses)
- Ice Cream
- Cream and Butter

Artificial Additives and Preservatives
- Artificial Sweeteners: Aspartame, saccharin, sucralose
- Preservatives: BHA, BHT, nitrites, nitrates
- Monosodium Glutamate (MSG)
- Artificial Colors and Flavors

Gluten (for those sensitive to it)
- Wheat-Based Products: Bread, pasta, pastries
- Barley
- Rye
- Certain Sauces and Soups (that contain wheat-based thickeners)

Alcohol
- Excessive Alcohol Consumption (can increase inflammation, especially when consumed in large amounts)

Trans Fats
- Hydrogenated Oils
- Processed Snack Foods
- Commercially Baked Goods: Cakes, cookies, pie crusts
- Microwave Popcorn (some brands)

High-Sodium Foods
- Canned Soups and Vegetables (unless labeled low-sodium
- Frozen Dinners
- Processed Snacks
- Fast Food

Certain Omega-6-Rich Foods
- Corn Oil
- Safflower Oil
- Soybean Oil
- Sunflower Oil (when consumed in excess, without balancing with omega-3s)

Excessive Red Meat
- Grain-Fed Beef and Pork (higher in inflammatory fats)

Processed Grains
- Instant Oatmeal
- White Flour Products
- Cornflakes

CHAPTER 4

QUICK AND EASY BREAKFASTS

Berry-Kefir Smoothie

Gluten-Free

Not Dairy-Free

Prep Time: 5 minutes Total Time: 5 minutes Serving Size: 1 smoothie (about 16 ounces)

Calories: 200

Fat: 7g

Protein: 8g

Carbs: 30g

Fiber: 8g

Sugars: 14g

- 1 cup mixed berries
- 1/2 cup plain kefir
- 1/2 cup unsweetened almond milk
- 1 tablespoon chia seeds
- 1/2 tablespoon honey or maple syrup (optional)
- 1/2 teaspoon ground turmeric
- 1/4 teaspoon ground cinnamon
- 1/4 teaspoon ground ginger
- A handful of spinach

Thoroughly wash the berries. Thawing frozen berries is not necessary if utilizing them.

Fill a blender with the following ingredients: spinach, berries, kefir, almond milk, chia seeds, honey, maple syrup, turmeric, cinnamon, ginger, and ginger.

Process the ingredients on high until it becomes creamy and smooth. To get the right consistency, thin down any extra smoothie by adding a little amount of almond milk.

Transfer to a glass.

Turmeric Latte

Gluten-Free: Yes

Dairy-Free: Yes

Vegan: Yes

Prep Time: 5 minutes **Cooking Time:** 5 minutes **Total Time:** 10 minutes **Serving Size:** 1 cup (about 8 ounces)

Calories: 120

Fat: 8g

Protein: 1g

Carbs: 11g

Fiber: 1g

Sugars: 7g

- 1 cup unsweetened almond milk
- 1/2 teaspoon ground turmeric
- 1/4 teaspoon ground cinnamon
- 1/4 teaspoon ground ginger
- A pinch of black pepper
- 1 teaspoon coconut oil or ghee
- 1 teaspoon honey or maple syrup

Warm, but not boiling, almond milk should be heated in a small saucepan over medium heat.

Incorporate the ginger, cinnamon, turmeric, and black pepper into the heated milk. Stirring constantly will help avoid clumping.

If using, stir in the ghee or coconut oil and honey or maple syrup until well mixed.

To let the flavors to merge, lower the heat to low and simmer the mixture for three to five minutes.

You may give the latte a brief blender run to get a frother texture.

Warm up the turmeric latte by pouring it into a cup.

Mango-Kale Smoothie

Gluten-Free: Yes

Dairy-Free: Yes   **Prep Time:** 5 minutes **Serving Size:** 1 smoothie (about 16 ounces)

Vegan: Yes

1 cup fresh or frozen mango chunks

1 tablespoon chia seeds

1/2 cup chopped kale (remove tough stems)

1/2 teaspoon ground turmeric

Calories: 190

1/2 banana

1/2 teaspoon grated ginger

Fat: 5g

A squeeze of fresh lime juice

1/2 cup unsweetened almond milk

Protein: 3g

1/2 cup water or coconut water

Carbs: 37g

Fiber: 7g

Sugars: 25g

If using fresh mango, peel and chop into chunks. Wash and chop the kale, removing the tough stems.

Add all the ingredients (mango, kale, banana, almond milk, water or coconut water, chia seeds, turmeric, ginger, and lime juice) to a blender.

Blend on high until the mixture is smooth and creamy. Add more water if needed to reach your desired consistency.

Pour into a glass

Cherry-Mocha Smoothie

Gluten-Free: Yes

Dairy-Free: Yes

Vegan: Yes

Prep Time: 5 minutes **Serving Size:** 1 smoothie (about 16 ounces)

- 1 cup frozen cherries
- 1/2 cup unsweetened almond milk or any plant-based milk of choice
- 1/2 cup brewed coffee, cooled
- 1 tablespoon unsweetened cocoa powder
- 1 tablespoon almond butter or any nut/seed butter of choice
- 1/2 tablespoon maple syrup
- 1/2 teaspoon vanilla extract
- 1/2 small beetroot, cooked and peeled

Calories: 200

Fat: 9g

Protein: 5g

Carbs: 29g

Fiber: 6g

Sugars: 17g

If using raw beetroot, cook and peel it beforehand.

Add all the ingredients (frozen cherries, almond milk, coffee, cocoa powder, almond butter, maple syrup, vanilla extract, and beetroot) to a blender.

Blend on high until the mixture is smooth and creamy. If the smoothie is too thick, add a bit more almond milk or coffee to reach your desired consistency.

Pour into a glass

Golden Milk

Gluten-Free: Yes

Dairy-Free: Yes

Vegan: Yes

Prep Time: 5 minutes Cooking Time: 5 minutes Total Time: 10 minutes Serving Size: 1 cup (about 8 ounces)

Calories: 130

Fat: 9g

Protein: 1g

Carbs: 12g

Fiber: 1g

Sugars: 7g

1 cup unsweetened coconut milk

1/2 teaspoon ground turmeric

1/4 teaspoon ground cinnamon

1/4 teaspoon ground ginger

A pinch of black pepper

1/2 teaspoon vanilla extract

1 teaspoon coconut oil

1 teaspoon maple syrup or honey

In a small saucepan, heat the coconut milk over medium heat until warm but not boiling.

Stir in the turmeric, cinnamon, ginger, and black pepper. Continue stirring until the spices are well mixed.

Add the vanilla extract, coconut oil, and maple syrup or honey, stirring until everything is fully combined.

Reduce the heat to low and let the mixture simmer for 3-5 minutes to allow the flavors to blend.

For a frothy texture, blend the golden milk in a blender for a few seconds.

Pour the golden milk into a mug and enjoy it warm.

Avocado-Banana Smoothie

Gluten-Free: Yes

Dairy-Free: Yes

Vegan: Yes

Prep Time: 5 minutes Serving Size: 1 smoothie (about 16 ounces)

- 1/2 ripe avocado
- 1 ripe banana
- 1 cup unsweetened almond milk
- 1 tablespoon chia seeds
- 1/2 tablespoon honey or maple syrup
- 1/2 teaspoon ground turmeric
- 1/4 teaspoon ground cinnamon
- 1/4 teaspoon ground ginger
- A handful of spinach

Calories: 280

Fat: 14g

Protein: 4g

Carbs: 38g

Fiber: 9g

Sugars: 17g

Scoop out the flesh of the avocado and peel the banana.

Add the avocado, banana, almond milk, chia seeds, honey/maple syrup, turmeric, cinnamon, ginger, and spinach (if using) to a blender.

Blend on high until the mixture is smooth and creamy. If the smoothie is too thick, add a little more almond milk to reach your desired consistency.

Pour into a glass

Beetroot Smoothie

Gluten-Free: Yes

Dairy-Free: Yes

Vegan: Yes

Prep Time: 10 minutes Serving Size: 1 smoothie (about 16 ounces)

Calories: 180

Fat: 4g

Protein: 3g

Carbohydrates: 36g

Fiber: 7g

Sugars: 20g

- 1 small raw beetroot, peeled and chopped
- 1/2 cup frozen mixed berries
- 1/2 banana, sliced
- 1/2 cup unsweetened almond milk
- 1/4 cup orange juice freshly squeezed if possible
- 1 tablespoon chia seeds
- 1/2 teaspoon ground ginger
- 1/2 teaspoon ground cinnamon
- 1/2 teaspoon turmeric powder
- 1 teaspoon honey or maple syrup

Peel and chop the beetroot. If you're using fresh berries, you might want to add a few ice cubes to make the smoothie cold.

Add the beetroot, mixed berries, banana, almond milk, orange juice, chia seeds, ginger, cinnamon, turmeric, and honey/maple syrup (if using) to a blender.

Blend on high until the mixture is smooth and creamy. If the smoothie is too thick, add a little more almond milk or orange juice to reach your desired consistency.

Pour into a glass

Pineapple-Ginger Smoothie

Gluten-Free: Yes

Dairy-Free: Yes

Vegan: Yes

Prep Time: 5 minutes Serving Size: 1 smoothie (about 16 ounces)

Calories: 150

Fat: 4g

Protein: 2g

Carbs: 30g

Fiber: 5g

Sugars: 18g

1 cup fresh or frozen pineapple chunks

1/2 cup unsweetened coconut water or water

1/2 cup unsweetened almond milk

1 tablespoon fresh ginger, peeled and grated

1/2 banana

1 tablespoon chia seeds

1 teaspoon honey or maple syrup

A handful of spinach

If using fresh pineapple, peel, core, and chop it into chunks. Peel and grate the ginger.

Add the pineapple, coconut water, almond milk, ginger, banana (if using), chia seeds, and sweetener to a blender.

Blend on high until the mixture is smooth and creamy. If the smoothie is too thick, add a little more coconut water or almond milk to reach your desired consistency.

Pour into a glass

Blueberry-Spinach Smoothie

Gluten-Free: Yes

Dairy-Free: Yes

Vegan: Yes

Prep Time: 5 minutes Serving Size: 1 smoothie (about 16 ounces)

Calories: 220

Fat: 8g

Protein: 5g

Carbohydrates: 30g

Fiber: 8g

Sugars: 17g

- 1 cup fresh or frozen blueberries
- 1 cup fresh spinach
- 1/2 cup unsweetened almond milk
- 1/2 cup plain coconut yogurt or any dairy-free yogurt
- 1 tablespoon chia seeds
- 1 teaspoon flax seeds
- 1/2 tablespoon maple syrup or honey
- 1/4 teaspoon ground turmeric
- 1/2 teaspoon vanilla extract

If using frozen blueberries, there is no need to thaw them. Wash the spinach if it's not pre-washed.

Add all the ingredients (blueberries, spinach, almond milk, coconut yogurt, chia seeds, flaxseeds, maple syrup/honey, turmeric, and vanilla extract) to a blender.

Blend on high until the mixture is smooth and creamy. If the smoothie is too thick, add a bit more almond milk to reach your desired consistency.

Pour into a glass

Spinach & Egg Scramble

Gluten-Free: Yes

Dairy-Free: No

Vegan: No

Prep Time: 5 minutes **Cooking Time:** 10 minutes **Total Time:** 15 minutes **Serving Size:** 1 serving

Calories: 240

Fat: 18g

Protein: 14g

Carbohydrates: 8g

Fiber: 2g

Sugars: 3g

- 2 large eggs
- 1 cup fresh spinach, chopped
- 1/4 cup diced onion
- 1/4 cup diced bell pepper (any color)
- 1 tablespoon olive oil
- Salt and pepper to taste
- 1/4 teaspoon ground turmeric
- 1 tablespoon nutritional yeast

Wash and chop the spinach. Dice the onion and bell pepper.

In a non-stick skillet, heat olive oil over medium heat.

Add the diced onion and bell pepper to the skillet. Sauté for about 3-4 minutes until they become soft.

Add the chopped spinach to the skillet and cook for an additional 1-2 minutes until wilted.

In a bowl, whisk the eggs with a pinch of salt, pepper, and ground turmeric (if using). Pour the egg mixture over the vegetables in the skillet.

Allow the eggs to cook undisturbed for about 1 minute, then gently stir and scramble until fully cooked, about 3-4 minutes.

If using, sprinkle the nutritional yeast over the scramble and stir to

combine.

Transfer to a plate and serve warm.

Green Smoothie

Gluten-Free: Yes

Dairy-Free: Yes

Vegan: Yes

Prep Time: 5 minutes Serving Size: 1 smoothie (about 16 ounces)

Calories: 280

Fat: 15g

Protein: 4g

Carbohydrates: 30g

Fiber: 10g

Sugars: 14g

1 cup spinach leaves (fresh or frozen)

1/2 cup kale leaves, stems removed, fresh or frozen

1 small green apple, cored and chopped

1/2 cucumber, peeled and chopped

1/2 avocado

1 tablespoon chia seeds

1 cup unsweetened almond milk

Juice of 1/2 lemon

1/2 teaspoon fresh ginger (grated) or 1/4 teaspoon ground ginger

1/2 cup water

1/2 tablespoon honey or maple syrup

Wash and chop the spinach, kale, apple, and cucumber. If using fresh ginger, grate it.

Add all the ingredients (spinach, kale, apple, cucumber, avocado, chia seeds, almond milk, lemon juice, ginger, and honey/maple syrup) to a blender.

Blend on high until the mixture is smooth and creamy. Add water as needed to adjust the consistency.

Pour into a glass

Avocado & Kale Omelet

Gluten-Free: Yes

Dairy-Free: No

Vegan: No

Prep Time: 10 minutes Cooking Time: 10 minutes Total Time: 20 minutes Serving Size: 1 omelet (about 2 eggs)

Calories: 300

Fat: 24g

Protein: 12g

Carbohydrates: 10g

Fiber: 6g

Sugars: 2g

2 large eggs

1/2 avocado, sliced

1/2 cup fresh kale, chopped

1 tablespoon olive oil or coconut oil

1/4 teaspoon garlic powder

1/4 teaspoon onion powder

Salt and pepper

Wash and chop the kale. Slice the avocado.

In a non-stick skillet, heat the olive oil or coconut oil over medium heat.

Add the chopped kale to the skillet and cook for about 2-3 minutes, or until wilted and slightly crispy.

In a bowl, beat the eggs with garlic powder, onion powder, salt, and pepper.

Pour the beaten eggs into the skillet over the kale. Let the eggs cook undisturbed for about 2-3 minutes, or until the edges start to set.

Carefully place the avocado slices on one half of the omelet.

Once the omelet is mostly set, fold it in half over the avocado. Cook

for another 1-2 minutes until the eggs are fully set.

Slide the omelet onto a plate and enjoy it warm..

Egg Salad Avocado Toast

Gluten-Free: No

Dairy-Free: Yes

Vegan: No

Prep Time: 10 minutes Cooking Time: 10 minutes Total Time: 20 minutes Serving Size: 1 slice of toast with egg salad

Calories: 350

Fat: 22g

Protein: 14g

Carbs: 30g

Fiber: 8g

Sugars: 4g

For the Egg Salad:

4 large eggs

2 tablespoons avocado mayonnaise or regular mayonnaise if preferred

1 tablespoon Dijon mustard

1 tablespoon chopped fresh dill or 1 teaspoon dried dill

1 tablespoon chopped chives or green onions

Salt and pepper

For the Toast:

1 slice of whole grain bread

1 ripe avocado

A squeeze of lemon juice

Salt and pepper

Cook the Eggs:

Place the eggs in a saucepan and cover with water.

Bring to a boil over medium-high heat, then cover and reduce heat to low. Simmer for 10 minutes.

Remove the eggs and place them in an ice bath or under cold running water to cool. Once cool, peel and chop the eggs.

Prepare the Egg Salad:

In a mixing bowl, combine the chopped eggs, avocado mayonnaise, Dijon mustard, dill, and chives. Mix well.

Season with salt and pepper to taste.

Prepare the Toast:

Toast the slice of bread to your desired level of crispness.

While the bread is toasting, mash the avocado in a small bowl and mix in the lemon juice, salt, and pepper.

Assemble the Toast:

Spread the mashed avocado evenly on the toasted bread.

Top with a generous portion of egg salad.

Garnish with additional chives or dill if desired.

Smoked Salmon & Omelet

Gluten-Free: Yes

Dairy-Free: No

Prep Time: 5 minutes Cooking Time: 5 minutes Total Time: 10 minutes Serving Size: 1 omelet

2 large eggs

1 tablespoon cream cheese regular or dairy-free alternative

2 ounces smoked salmon

Calories: 300

1 tablespoon chopped fresh dill or chives

Fat: 22g

1 tablespoon olive oil or butter

Protein: 21g

Salt and pepper

Carbs: 2g

Fiber: 0g

Sugars: 1g

Beat the eggs in a bowl and season with salt and pepper. Chop the smoked salmon into bite-sized pieces.

Heat the olive oil or butter in a non-stick skillet over medium heat.

Pour the beaten eggs into the skillet and let them cook undisturbed until the edges start to set, about 2-3 minutes.

Spread the cream cheese evenly over one half of the omelet. Add the smoked salmon and dill on top of the cream cheese.

Carefully fold the omelet in half over the filling. Cook for an additional 1-2 minutes, until the omelet is cooked through and the cheese is melted.

Slide the omelet onto a plate and serve warm.

Southwestern Waffle with Eggs

Gluten-Free: Yes

Dairy-Free: No

Vegan: No

Prep Time: 10 minutes Cooking Time: 15 minutes Total Time: 25 minutes Serving Size: 1 waffle with 2 eggs

Calories: 400

Fat: 22g

Protein: 17g

Carbs: 37g

Fiber: 7g

Sugars: 6g

For the Waffle:

1 cup gluten-free waffle mix

1/2 cup water or as required by waffle mix instructions

1 tablespoon coconut oil or melted ghee

For the Toppings:

2 large eggs

1/4 cup shredded cheddar cheese

1/4 cup black beans, rinsed and drained

- 1/4 cup diced tomatoes

1/4 avocado, sliced

2 tablespoons fresh cilantro, chopped

1/4 teaspoon ground cumin

Salt and pepper to taste

In a bowl, mix the gluten-free waffle mix with water and coconut oil according to the package instructions. Preheat the waffle maker.

Pour the batter into the preheated waffle maker and cook according to the manufacturer's instructions until golden brown and crispy. Remove and set aside.

While the waffle is cooking, heat a non-stick skillet over medium heat. Crack the eggs into the skillet and cook until the whites are set and the yolks are cooked to your preference. Season with salt and pepper.

Place the cooked waffle on a plate. Top with shredded cheese (if using), black beans, diced tomatoes, and avocado slices.

Place the cooked eggs on top of the waffle. Sprinkle with ground cumin and chopped cilantro.

Enjoy while warm.

Egg & Veggie Burrito

Gluten-Free: Yes

Dairy-Free: Yes

Vegan: No

Prep Time: 10 minutes Cooking Time: 15 minutes Total Time: 25 minutes Serving Size: 1 burrito

Calories: 350

Fat: 20g

Protein: 15g

Carbs: 30g

Fiber: 6g

Sugars: 5g

- 1 gluten-free tortilla (or any tortilla of choice)
- 2 large eggs
- 1/2 cup diced bell peppers (any color)
- 1/2 cup chopped spinach
- 1/4 cup diced onion
- 1/4 cup diced tomatoes
- 1 tablespoon olive oil or avocado oil
- 1/4 teaspoon ground turmeric
- 1/4 teaspoon ground black pepper
- 1/4 teaspoon ground cumin
- 1/4 teaspoon paprika
- Salt
- 1 tablespoon dairy-free cheese or regular cheese

Dice the bell peppers, onion, and tomatoes. Chop the spinach.

In a skillet, heat the olive oil over medium heat. Add the onion and bell peppers and sauté for 3-4 minutes until softened. Add the tomatoes and spinach, and cook for an additional 2 minutes. Season with turmeric, black pepper, cumin, paprika, and salt. Remove from heat and set aside.

In a bowl, whisk the eggs. Pour them into the same skillet and cook over medium heat, stirring occasionally, until fully cooked. Combine with the vegetable mixture.

Warm the tortilla according to package instructions. Place the egg and veggie mixture in the center of the tortilla. If using, sprinkle dairy-free cheese or regular cheese over the top.

Fold in the sides of the tortilla and roll it up to form a burrito.

Mushroom & Spinach Frittata

Gluten-Free: Yes

Dairy-Free: Yes

Vegan: No

Prep Time: 10 minutes Cooking Time: 20 minutes Total Time: 30 minutes Serving Size: 1 slice (1/8 of the frittata)

Calories: 160

Fat: 11g

Protein: 12g

Carbs: 4g

Fiber: 1g

Sugars: 2g

6 large eggs

1 cup mushrooms, sliced

1 cup fresh spinach, chopped

1/2 small onion, finely chopped

2 cloves garlic, minced

1 tablespoon olive oil

1/4 teaspoon ground turmeric

1/4 teaspoon ground black pepper

1/4 teaspoon dried thyme

Salt

Preheat your oven to 375°F (190°C).

In an oven-safe skillet, heat the olive oil over medium heat. Add the onions and garlic, and sauté until softened, about 3-4 minutes.

Add the mushrooms to the skillet and cook until they release their moisture and start to brown, about 5 minutes.

Stir in the spinach and cook until wilted, about 2 minutes. Season with turmeric, black pepper, thyme, and salt.

In a bowl, whisk the eggs until well beaten. Pour the eggs over the vegetable mixture in the skillet, making sure they are evenly distributed.

Let the frittata cook on the stovetop for about 2-3 minutes, until the edges start to set.

Transfer the skillet to the preheated oven and bake for 15-20 minutes,

or until the frittata is set in the middle and lightly golden on top.

Allow the frittata to cool slightly before slicing and serving.

Banana Oat Pancakes

Gluten-Free: Yes

Dairy-Free: Yes

Vegan: Yes

Prep Time: 10 minutes Cooking Time: 15 minutes Total Time: 25 minutes Serving Size: 2 pancakes (about 4 inches in diameter each)

(per serving, 2 pancakes):

Calories: 180

Fat: 5g

Protein: 5g

Carbs: 30g

Fiber: 4g

Sugars: 9g

- 1 ripe banana
- 1 cup rolled oats (use gluten-free oats if needed)
- 1/2 cup almond milk or any plant-based milk
- 1 tablespoon ground flaxseed
- 1/2 teaspoon baking powder
- 1/2 teaspoon ground cinnamon
- 1/4 teaspoon vanilla extract
- Coconut oil or non-stick spray

In a blender, combine the banana, oats, almond milk, ground flaxseed, baking powder, cinnamon, and vanilla extract. Blend until smooth.

Heat a non-stick skillet or griddle over medium heat. Lightly grease with coconut oil or non-stick spray.

Pour 1/4 cup of batter onto the skillet for each pancake. Cook for 2-3 minutes or until bubbles form on the surface. Flip and cook for another 1-2 minutes until golden brown.

Serve warm with your favorite toppings, such as fresh fruit, a drizzle of maple syrup, or a sprinkle of nuts.

Sweet Potato Waffles

Gluten-Free: Yes

Dairy-Free: Yes

Vegan: Yes

Prep Time: 10 minutes Cooking Time: 15 minutes Total Time: 25 minutes Serving Size: 1 waffle (about 1/2 cup batter per waffle)

Calories: 160

Fat: 10g

Protein: 4g

Carbs: 18g

Fiber: 4g

Sugars: 6g

- 1 large sweet potato, peeled and cubed
- 1/2 cup almond flour
- 1/4 cup coconut flour
- 2 tablespoons flaxseed meal
- 1/2 teaspoon baking powder
- 1/2 teaspoon ground cinnamon
- 1/4 teaspoon ground nutmeg
- 1/4 teaspoon salt
- 1/4 cup unsweetened almond milk
- 2 tablespoons maple syrup or honey
- 1 tablespoon coconut oil

Boil or steam the sweet potato cubes until tender, about 10 minutes. Drain and let cool slightly.

Mash the sweet potato in a bowl until smooth.

In a separate bowl, mix the almond flour, coconut flour, flaxseed meal, baking powder, cinnamon, nutmeg, and salt.

Add the mashed sweet potato, almond milk, maple syrup (if using), and coconut oil to the dry ingredients. Stir until well combined.

Preheat your waffle iron according to the manufacturer's instructions.

Lightly grease the waffle iron with a bit of oil or cooking spray. Pour about 1/2 cup of batter into the waffle iron and cook until the waffles are golden brown and crisp, about 4-5 minutes.

Remove from the waffle iron and serve warm with your favorite toppings.

Pumpkin Spice Pancakes

Gluten-Free: Yes

Dairy-Free: Yes

Vegan: Yes

Prep Time: 10 minutes Cooking Time: 15 minutes Total Time: 25 minutes Serving Size: 2 pancakes

1 cup gluten-free all-purpose flour or regular flour if not required to be gluten-free

1/2 cup canned pumpkin puree (pure pumpkin, not pumpkin pie filling)

1/2 cup unsweetened almond milk

(per serving of 2 pancakes):

1 tablespoon maple syrup

Calories: 220

1 teaspoon ground cinnamon

Fat: 10g

1/2 teaspoon ground nutmeg

Protein: 4g

1/4 teaspoon ground ginger

1/2 teaspoon baking powder

1/4 teaspoon baking soda

A pinch of salt

1 tablespoon coconut oil

In a large bowl, whisk together the flour, baking powder, baking soda, cinnamon, nutmeg, ginger, and salt.

In another bowl, mix the pumpkin puree, almond milk, maple syrup, and 1 tablespoon of coconut oil until well combined.

Pour the wet ingredients into the dry ingredients and stir until just combined. The batter should be slightly lumpy.

Heat a non-stick skillet or griddle over medium heat. Add a small amount of coconut oil to coat the surface.

Pour 1/4 cup of batter onto the skillet for each pancake. Cook until bubbles form on the surface, then flip and cook until golden brown on the other side, about 2-3 minutes per side.

Serve warm with your favorite toppings.

Lemon-Blueberry Ricotta Pancakes

Gluten-Free: No

Dairy-Free: No

Vegan: No

Prep Time: 10 minutes **Cooking Time:** 15 minutes **Total Time:** 25 minutes **Serving Size:** 2 pancakes

- 1/2 cup ricotta cheese
- 1/2 cup all-purpose flour (for gluten-free, use a gluten-free flour blend)
- 1/4 cup almond flour
- 1/4 cup milk
- 1 large egg
- 1 tablespoon honey or maple syrup
- 1 teaspoon lemon zest
- 1 tablespoon lemon juice
- 1/2 teaspoon baking powder
- 1/4 teaspoon salt
- 1/2 cup fresh blueberries
- 1 tablespoon coconut oil or butter

(per serving, 2 pancakes):

Calories: 280

Fat: 14g

Protein: 10g

Carbohydrates: 31g

Fiber: 3g

Sugars: 11g

In a mixing bowl, combine the ricotta cheese, flour, almond flour, milk, egg, honey or maple syrup, lemon zest, lemon juice, baking powder, and salt. Mix until just combined.

Gently fold in the blueberries.

Heat a non-stick skillet or griddle over medium heat and add coconut oil or butter.

Pour 1/4 cup of batter onto the skillet for each pancake. Cook for 2-3 minutes on each side, or until golden brown and cooked through.

Serve warm with extra blueberries and a drizzle of honey or maple syrup if desired.

Chia Seed Pancakes

Gluten-Free: Yes

Dairy-Free: Yes

Vegan: Yes

Prep Time: 10 minutes Cooking Time: 15 minutes Total Time: 25 minutes Serving Size: 2 pancakes

1/2 cup chia seeds

1 cup unsweetened almond milk or any plant-based milk of choice

1 tablespoon maple syrup or honey

1 cup gluten-free flour blend

1 tablespoon baking powder

1/2 teaspoon vanilla extract

1/4 teaspoon salt

2 tablespoons flaxseed meal mixed with 6 tablespoons water (flax egg substitute)

(per serving of 2 pancakes):

Calories: 200

Fat: 8g

Protein: 6g

Carbs: 30g

Fiber: 8g

Sugars: 5g

Mix chia seeds with almond milk and let sit for about 5 minutes until they form a gel-like consistency.

In a small bowl, mix flaxseed meal with water and let sit for a few minutes to thicken.

In a large bowl, whisk together the gluten-free flour blend, baking powder, and salt.

Add the chia seed mixture, flax egg, vanilla extract, and maple syrup or honey to the dry ingredients. Stir until well combined.

Heat a non-stick skillet or griddle over medium heat and lightly grease with coconut oil or cooking spray.

Pour about 1/4 cup of batter per pancake onto the skillet. Cook for 2-3 minutes on each side or until bubbles form on the surface and the edges look set.

Remove from the skillet and serve warm with your favorite toppings.

CHAPTER 5

SNACKS AND HAPPY BITES

Turmeric Roasted Chickpeas

Gluten-Free: Yes

Dairy-Free: Yes

Vegan: Yes

Prep Time: 10 minutes Cooking Time: 30 minutes Total Time: 40 minutes Serving Size: 1/4 cup (about 40 grams)

(per serving, 1/4 cup):

Calories: 120

Fat: 6g

Protein: 5g

Carbs: 14g

Fiber: 4g

Sugars: 2g

- 1 can (15 oz) chickpeas, drained and rinsed
- 1 tablespoon olive oil
- 1/2 teaspoon ground turmeric
- 1/2 teaspoon ground cumin
- 1/4 teaspoon smoked paprika
- 1/4 teaspoon garlic powder
- 1/4 teaspoon onion powder
- Salt and black pepper

Preheat your oven to 400°F (200°C).

Pat the chickpeas dry with a towel to remove excess moisture.

In a large bowl, toss the chickpeas with olive oil, turmeric, cumin, smoked paprika, garlic powder, onion powder, salt, and black pepper until evenly coated.

Spread the chickpeas in a single layer on a baking sheet. Roast for 25-30 minutes, stirring halfway through, until they are crispy and golden brown.

Allow the chickpeas to cool before serving. They will become crunchier as they cool.

Avocado Hummus

Gluten-Free: Yes

Dairy-Free: Yes

Vegan: Yes

Prep Time: 10 minutes Serving Size: 1/4 cup (about 60 grams)

1 ripe avocado

1 can (15 oz) chickpeas, drained and rinsed

1/4 cup tahini

2 tablespoons fresh lemon juice

1 garlic clove, minced

1/4 teaspoon ground cumin

Salt

2-3 tablespoons water

A pinch of paprika

Calories: 100

Fat: 6g

Protein: 4g

Carbs: 9g

Fiber: 4g

Sugars: 1g

Scoop the avocado flesh into a food processor.

Add the chickpeas, tahini, lemon juice, garlic, cumin, and salt.

Process until smooth, scraping down the sides as needed. Add water a little at a time until the hummus reaches your desired consistency.

Taste and adjust salt or lemon juice as needed.

Transfer to a bowl and sprinkle with paprika if desired. Serve with vegetable sticks, pita, or as a spread.

Nut Butter Apple Slices

Gluten-Free: Yes

Dairy-Free: Yes **Prep Time:** 5 minutes **Serving Size:** 1 apple, sliced (about 8 slices)

Vegan: Yes

1 large apple

2 tablespoons almond butter or peanut butter, make sure it's unsweetened and contains no added sugar or dairy

A sprinkle of cinnamon

(per serving, 8 slices): A few chia seeds or granola

Calories: 200

Fat: 14g

Core and slice the apple into thin, even slices.

Protein: 4g

Spread a tablespoon of almond butter or peanut butter evenly over each apple slice.

Carbohydrates: 20g

Fiber: 4g

Sprinkle with cinnamon, chia seeds, or granola if desired.

Sugars: 14g

Arrange the slices on a plate

Cucumber and Hummus Bites

Gluten-Free: Yes

Dairy-Free: Yes

Vegan: Yes

Prep Time: 10 minutes Serving Size: 4 bites (about 4 ounces)

1 large cucumber

1/2 cup hummus (store-bought or homemade)

1 tablespoon chopped fresh parsley

1 tablespoon sliced black olives

1/2 teaspoon ground paprika

Salt and pepper

(per serving, 4 bites):

Calories: 80

Fat: 5g

Protein: 2g

Carbohydrates: 7g

Fiber: 2g

Sugars: 3g

Wash and peel the cucumber (optional). Slice it into 1/4-inch thick rounds.

Spread a small amount of hummus on each cucumber slice.

Sprinkle with chopped parsley, sliced black olives (if using), paprika, and a pinch of salt and pepper.

Arrange the cucumber bites on a serving plate

Golden Milk Energy Balls

Gluten-Free: Yes

Dairy-Free: Yes

Vegan: Yes

Prep Time: 10 minutes Serving Size: 1 energy ball (makes about 12 balls)

1 cup rolled oats (use certified gluten-free oats if needed)

1/2 cup almond flour

1/4 cup shredded unsweetened coconut

1/4 cup almond butter or cashew butter

1/4 cup pure maple syrup or honey

1 tablespoon ground turmeric

1/2 teaspoon ground cinnamon

1/2 teaspoon ground ginger

1/4 teaspoon black pepper

1 tablespoon chia seeds

(per serving, 1 ball):

Calories: 90

Fat: 6g

Protein: 2g

Carbohydrates: 9g

Fiber: 2g

Sugars: 5g

In a large bowl, combine the rolled oats, almond flour, shredded coconut, ground turmeric, cinnamon, ginger, and black pepper. Stir in the chia seeds if using.

In a separate bowl, mix the almond butter and maple syrup or honey until smooth.

Add the wet ingredients to the dry ingredients and mix until well combined. The mixture should be slightly sticky and hold together when pressed.

Roll the mixture into small balls, about 1 inch in diameter. If the mixture is too sticky, lightly dampen your hands with water.

Place the energy balls on a parchment-lined baking sheet or plate.

Refrigerate for at least 30 minutes to firm up.

Enjoy chilled or at room temperature. Store leftovers in an airtight container in the fridge for up to 1 week.

Carrot and Celery Sticks with Guacamole

Gluten-Free: Yes

Dairy-Free: Yes

Vegan: Yes

Prep Time: 10 minutes Serving Size: 1 serving (about 1 cup of guacamole with vegetable sticks)

(per serving, including about 1/2 cup guacamole and vegetable sticks):

Calories: 150

Fat: 10g

Protein: 2g

Carbs: 15g

Fiber: 7g

Sugars: 6g

For the Guacamole:

2 ripe avocados

1 small tomato, diced

1/4 cup red onion, finely chopped

1 clove garlic, minced

1 tablespoon lime juice

1/4 teaspoon ground cumin

1/4 teaspoon ground turmeric

Salt and pepper

For the Vegetable Sticks:

2 large carrots, peeled and cut into sticks

2 celery stalks, cut into sticks

Prepare the Guacamole:

In a bowl, scoop out the flesh of the avocados and mash with a fork until smooth but still slightly chunky.

Add the diced tomato, red onion, garlic, lime juice, cumin, turmeric, salt, and pepper.

Mix until all ingredients are well combined. Adjust seasoning to taste.

Prepare the Vegetable Sticks:

Peel and cut the carrots into sticks.

Wash and cut the celery stalks into sticks.

Serve:

Arrange the carrot and celery sticks on a plate or serving dish.

Serve alongside a bowl of guacamole for dipping.

Blueberry Almond Bites

Gluten-Free: Yes

Dairy-Free: Yes

Vegan: Yes

Prep Time: 15 minutes Serving Size: 4 bites and 1/4 cup guacamole

(per serving, 4 bites with 1/4 cup guacamole):

Blueberry Almond Bites:

Calories (per bite): 60 kcal

Fat (per bite): 5g

Protein (per bite): 2g

Carbs (per bite): 5g

Fiber (per bite): 2g

Sugars (per bite): 2g

Guacamole:

Calories (per 1/4 cup): 100

Fat (per 1/4 cup): 9g

Protein (per 1/4 cup):

For the Blueberry Almond Bites:

1 cup almonds

1/2 cup dried blueberries (unsweetened)

2 tablespoons chia seeds

1 tablespoon honey or maple syrup

1/2 teaspoon vanilla extract

For the Guacamole:

1 ripe avocado

1 tablespoon lime juice

1/4 teaspoon garlic powder

1/4 teaspoon onion powder

A pinch of salt

1 tablespoon finely chopped cilantro

1/4 cup diced tomatoes

For the Blueberry Almond Bites:

In a food processor, combine the almonds and dried blueberries. Process until the mixture is finely chopped and begins to stick together.

Add the chia seeds, honey or maple syrup, and vanilla extract. Process until well mixed and the mixture holds together when pressed.

Roll the mixture into small balls, about 1 inch in diameter. Place them on a plate or tray.

Refrigerate the bites for at least 15 minutes to firm up.

1g

Carbohydrates (per 1/4 cup): 6g

Fiber (per 1/4 cup): 4g

Sugars (per 1/4 cup): 1g

For the Guacamole:

In a bowl, mash the avocado with a fork until smooth.

Add lime juice, garlic powder, onion powder, salt, cilantro (if using), and diced tomatoes (if using). Mix until well combined.

Serve the guacamole with the blueberry almond bites.

Sweet Potato Chips

Gluten-Free: Yes

Dairy-Free: Yes

Vegan: Yes

Prep Time: 15 minutes Cooking Time: 25-30 minutes Total Time: 40-45 minutes Serving Size: About 1 ounce (28 grams)

2 large sweet potatoes

1-2 tablespoons olive oil

1/2 teaspoon paprika

1/2 teaspoon garlic powder

1/2 teaspoon onion powder

1/4 teaspoon sea salt

(per serving of 1 ounce or 28 grams):

1/4 teaspoon black pepper

Calories: 130

Fat: 7g

Protein: 1g

Carbs: 18g

Fiber: 3g

Sugars: 6g

Preheat your oven to 400°F (200°C).

Wash and peel the sweet potatoes. Slice them thinly (about 1/8 inch thick) using a mandolin or sharp knife.

In a large bowl, toss the sweet potato slices with olive oil, paprika, garlic powder, onion powder, salt, and black pepper (if using) until evenly coated.

Spread the sweet potato slices in a single layer on a baking sheet lined with parchment paper. Avoid overlapping to ensure they crisp up evenly.

Bake for 25-30 minutes, flipping the slices halfway through, until the chips are crispy and golden brown. Keep an eye on them as baking times can vary.

Let the chips cool on a wire rack to maintain their crispiness.

Enjoy or store in an airtight container for up to 1 week.

Turmeric Popcorn

Gluten-Free: Yes

Dairy-Free: Yes

Vegan: Yes

Prep Time: 10 minutes Cooking Time: 10 minutes Total Time: 20 minutes Serving Size: 1 cup popped popcorn

1/2 cup popcorn kernels

1 tablespoon coconut oil or avocado oil

1/2 teaspoon ground turmeric

1/4 teaspoon ground cumin

1/4 teaspoon paprika

1/4 teaspoon garlic powder

1/4 teaspoon onion powder

Salt

(per serving, 1 cup popped popcorn):

Calories: 60

Fat: 3g

Protein: 2g

Carbs: 8g

Fiber: 2g

Sugars: 0g

Heat the coconut oil or avocado oil in a large pot over medium heat. Add a few popcorn kernels to test if the oil is hot enough. Once they pop, add the remaining popcorn kernels

Cover the pot with a lid, leaving a small gap for steam to escape. Shake the pot occasionally to ensure even popping and prevent burning.

Once popping slows down, remove the pot from heat. Transfer the popped popcorn to a large bowl. Immediately sprinkle the turmeric, cumin, paprika, garlic powder, onion powder, and salt over the popcorn while it's still warm. Toss well to coat evenly.

Enjoy the seasoned popcorn warm or let it cool before storing in an airtight container.

CHAPTER 6
SALADS, WRAPS AND SIDE DISHES

Kale and Quinoa Salad

Gluten-Free: Yes

Dairy-Free: Yes

Vegan: Yes

Prep Time: 15 minutes Cooking Time: 15 minutes Total Time: 30 minutes Serving Size: 1 cup

Calories: 250

Fat: 12g

Protein: 7g

Carbohydrates: 31g

Fiber: 5g

Sugars: 7g

For the Salad:

1 cup quinoa (uncooked)

2 cups water

4 cups chopped kale (stems removed)

1 cup cherry tomatoes, halved

1/2 cucumber, diced

1/4 cup red onion, finely chopped

1/4 cup sliced almonds

1/4 cup dried cranberries

For the Dressing:

3 tablespoons extra virgin olive oil

2 tablespoons lemon juice

1 tablespoon apple cider vinegar

1 teaspoon Dijon mustard

1 clove garlic, minced

Salt and pepper

Rinse the quinoa under cold water. In a medium saucepan, bring 2 cups of water to a boil. Add the quinoa, reduce heat to low, cover, and simmer for 15 minutes, or until water is absorbed and quinoa is tender. Fluff with a fork and let cool.

While the quinoa cooks, massage the chopped kale with a little bit of olive oil and a pinch of salt for about 1-2 minutes until it becomes tender.

In a small bowl, whisk together the olive oil, lemon juice, apple cider vinegar, Dijon mustard, minced garlic, salt, and pepper.

In a large bowl, combine the cooked quinoa, massaged kale, cherry tomatoes, cucumber, red onion, almonds, and cranberries.

Pour the dressing over the salad and toss to coat all ingredients evenly.

Chill in the refrigerator for 10-15 minutes before serving for best flavor.

Spinach and Berry Salad

Gluten-Free: Yes

Dairy-Free: Yes   Prep Time: 10 minutes Serving Size: 1 salad (about 2 cups)

Vegan: Yes

2 cups fresh spinach leaves

1/2 cup mixed berries

1/4 cup sliced almonds

1/4 cup crumbled feta cheese

1 tablespoon chia seeds

Calories: 220   1 tablespoon extra virgin olive oil

Fat: 14g   1 tablespoon balsamic vinegar

Protein: 6g   1 teaspoon honey or maple syrup

Carbs: 20g   Salt and pepper

Fiber: 6g

Sugars: 10g   Wash the spinach leaves and berries thoroughly. Pat dry with a paper towel.

In a large bowl, combine the spinach leaves, mixed berries, sliced almonds, and chia seeds.

In a small bowl, whisk together the olive oil, balsamic vinegar, honey or maple syrup, salt, and pepper.

Drizzle the dressing over the salad and toss gently to combine.

Divide the salad into bowls or plates

Turmeric Chickpea Salad

Gluten-Free: Yes

Dairy-Free: Yes

Vegan: Yes

Prep Time: 15 minutes Serving Size: 1 cup

- 1 can (15 oz) chickpeas, drained and rinsed (or 1.5 cups cooked chickpeas)
- 1/2 cup diced cucumber
- 1/2 cup cherry tomatoes, halved
- 1/4 cup red onion, finely chopped
- 1/4 cup fresh parsley, chopped
- 1 tablespoon olive oil
- 1 tablespoon lemon juice
- 1/2 teaspoon ground turmeric
- 1/4 teaspoon ground cumin
- 1/4 teaspoon paprika
- Salt and pepper

Calories: 180

Fat: 8g

Protein: 6g

Carbohydrates: 22g

Fiber: 6g

Sugars: 4g

Dice the cucumber, halve the cherry tomatoes, and finely chop the red onion and parsley.

In a large bowl, combine the chickpeas, cucumber, cherry tomatoes, red onion, and parsley.

In a small bowl, whisk together the olive oil, lemon juice, turmeric, cumin, paprika, salt, and pepper.

Pour the dressing over the salad and toss well to combine.

Chill for 10 minutes if desired, then serve.

Arugula and Beet Salad

Gluten-Free: Yes

Dairy-Free: Yes

Vegan: Yes

Prep Time: 15 minutes Cooking Time: 30 minutes Total Time: 45 minutes Serving Size: 1 serving (about 2 cups)

- 2 medium beets, peeled and cut into cubes
- 1 tablespoon olive oil
- Salt and pepper
- 4 cups fresh arugula
- 1/4 cup crumbled feta cheese
- 1/4 cup chopped walnuts
- 1/4 cup thinly sliced red onion
- 2 tablespoons balsamic vinegar
- 1 tablespoon honey or maple syrup

Calories: 250

Fat: 16g

Protein: 6g

Carbohydrates: 26g

Fiber: 6g

Sugars: 15g

Preheat the oven to 400°F (200°C). Toss the beet cubes with olive oil, salt, and pepper. Spread them on a baking sheet and roast for 25-30 minutes, or until tender. Allow to cool slightly.

While the beets are roasting, wash and dry the arugula. Place it in a large salad bowl.

Once the beets are cool, add them to the bowl with arugula. If using, sprinkle the crumbled feta cheese, chopped walnuts, and sliced red onion over the top.

In a small bowl, whisk together the balsamic vinegar and honey or maple syrup, if using. Adjust seasoning with salt and pepper.

Drizzle the dressing over the salad and toss gently to combine.

Serve or chill until ready to eat.

Mediterranean Lentil Salad

Gluten-Free: Yes

Dairy-Free: Yes

Vegan: Yes

Prep Time: 15 minutes Cooking Time: 25 minutes Total Time: 40 minutes Serving Size: 1 cup (about 200 grams)

(per serving, 1 cup):

Calories: 250

Fat: 12g

Protein: 10g

Carbohydrates: 29g

Fiber: 8g

Sugars: 4g

1 cup dried green or brown lentils

2 1/2 cups water

1 cup cherry tomatoes, halved

1/2 cup cucumber, diced

1/4 cup red onion, finely chopped

1/4 cup Kalamata olives, pitted and sliced

1/4 cup fresh parsley, chopped

1/4 cup fresh mint, chopped

1/4 cup extra-virgin olive oil

2 tablespoons lemon juice

1 teaspoon dried oregano

Salt and pepper

. Rinse the lentils under cold water. In a medium saucepan, combine lentils and water. Bring to a boil, then reduce heat and simmer for about 20-25 minutes, or until lentils are tender. Drain and let cool.

While lentils are cooking, prepare the cherry tomatoes, cucumber, red onion, olives, parsley, and mint.

In a small bowl, whisk together olive oil, lemon juice, oregano, salt, and pepper.

In a large bowl, combine the cooked lentils with the prepared vegetables and herbs. Pour the dressing over the salad and toss to combine.

Chill in the refrigerator for at least 30 minutes to let flavors meld. Serve cold or at room temperature.

Cauliflower Rice Salad

Gluten-Free: Yes

Dairy-Free: Yes

Vegan: Yes

Prep Time: 15 minutes Cooking Time: 10 minutes Total Time: 25 minutes Serving Size: 1 cup

Calories: 150 kcal

Fat: 8g

Protein: 3g

Carbs: 15g

Fiber: 5g

Sugars: 6g

1 medium head of cauliflower

1 tablespoon olive oil

1 cup cherry tomatoes, halved

1/2 cucumber, diced

1/4 red onion, finely chopped

1/4 cup fresh parsley, chopped

1/4 cup fresh basil, chopped

1/4 cup black olives, sliced

1 tablespoon lemon juice

1 tablespoon apple cider vinegar

Salt and pepper

Prepare Cauliflower Rice:

Remove the leaves and stem from the cauliflower and cut it into florets.

Use a food processor to pulse the florets into rice-sized pieces.

Heat olive oil in a large skillet over medium heat. Add the cauliflower rice and cook, stirring occasionally, for about 5-7 minutes until tender but not mushy. Let it cool.

In a large bowl, combine the cooked cauliflower rice, cherry tomatoes, cucumber, red onion, parsley, basil, and black olives.

In a small bowl, whisk together lemon juice, apple cider vinegar, salt, and pepper.

Pour the dressing over the salad and toss to coat evenly. Adjust seasoning if needed.

Sweet Potato and Black Bean Salad

Gluten-Free: Yes

Dairy-Free: Yes

Vegan: Yes

Prep Time: 15 minutes Cooking Time: 25 minutes Total Time: 40 minutes Serving Size: 1 cup

2 medium sweet potatoes, peeled and diced

1 tablespoon olive oil

1/2 teaspoon ground cumin

1/2 teaspoon smoked paprika

1/4 teaspoon salt

1/4 teaspoon black pepper

1 cup cooked black beans (canned, drained, and rinsed)

1/2 cup chopped red bell pepper

1/4 cup chopped red onion

1/4 cup fresh cilantro, chopped

2 tablespoons fresh lime juice

1 tablespoon extra virgin olive oil

Calories: 220

Fat: 7g

Protein: 8g

Carbohydrates: 32g

Fiber: 8g

Preheat your oven to 400°F (200°C).

Toss the diced sweet potatoes with 1 tablespoon of olive oil, cumin, smoked paprika, salt, and black pepper. Spread on a baking sheet in a single layer and roast for 20-25 minutes, or until tender and slightly caramelized, turning halfway through.

In a large bowl, combine the cooked sweet potatoes, black beans, red bell pepper, red onion, and cilantro.

In a small bowl, whisk together the lime juice and extra virgin olive oil.

Pour the dressing over the salad and toss gently to coat all ingredients evenly.

Chill for at least 10 minutes before serving to allow flavors to meld.

Chicken and Spinach Wrap

Gluten-Free: Yes

Dairy-Free: Yes

Vegan: No

Prep Time: 10 minutes Cooking Time: 10 minutes Total Time: 20 minutes Serving Size: 1 wrap

Calories: 350

Fat: 18g

Protein: 25g

Carbs: 30g

Fiber: 8g

Sugars: 4g

1 gluten-free wrap or tortilla or use a regular wrap if gluten is not a concern

4 ounces cooked chicken breast, sliced or shredded

1 cup fresh spinach leaves

1/4 avocado, sliced

1/4 cup shredded carrots

2 tablespoons hummus or any preferred spread

1 tablespoon olive oil

Salt and pepper

1 tablespoon dairy-free cheese or regular cheese

If not using pre-cooked chicken, season chicken breast with salt and pepper. Heat olive oil in a skillet over medium heat and cook chicken for about 6-7 minutes on each side, until fully cooked. Slice or shred once done.

Spread hummus evenly over the wrap.

Layer the spinach, avocado slices, shredded carrots, and cooked chicken on top of the hummus. Add dairy-free cheese if desired.

Fold in the sides of the wrap and then roll it up tightly from the bottom.

Cut the wrap in half if desired.

Tofu and Veggie Wrap

Gluten-Free: No

Dairy-Free: Yes

Vegan: Yes

Prep Time: 10 minutes Cooking Time: 15 minutes Total Time: 25 minutes Serving Size: 1 wrap

Calories: 300

Fat: 14g

Protein: 12g

Carbohydrates: 32g

Fiber: 6g

Sugars: 6g

- 1 large whole-grain or gluten-free wrap (8-10 inches)
- 1/2 cup extra-firm tofu, cubed
- 1 tablespoon olive oil
- 1/2 teaspoon ground turmeric
- 1/2 teaspoon ground cumin
- 1/4 teaspoon smoked paprika
- 1/4 teaspoon garlic powder
- 1/4 teaspoon onion powder
- Salt and pepper
- 1/2 cup shredded carrots
- 1/2 cup thinly sliced red bell pepper
- 1/2 cup baby spinach
- 1/4 cup hummus
- 1 tablespoon chopped fresh cilantro or parsley

In a bowl, toss the cubed tofu with olive oil, turmeric, cumin, smoked paprika, garlic powder, onion powder, salt, and pepper.

Heat a non-stick skillet over medium heat. Add the seasoned tofu and cook for 8-10 minutes, stirring occasionally, until golden and crispy on all sides.

While the tofu cooks, prepare the shredded carrots, sliced bell pepper, and baby spinach.

If using, spread a thin layer of hummus over the wrap. Lay down the cooked tofu and top with shredded carrots, bell pepper, and spinach.

Roll the wrap tightly, slice in half if desired, and garnish with fresh

cilantro or parsley if using.

Garlic Green Beans

Gluten-Free: Yes

Dairy-Free: Yes

Vegan: Yes

Prep Time: 10 minutes Cooking Time: 10 minutes Total Time: 20 minutes Serving Size: 1 cup (about 130 grams)

1 pound (450 grams) fresh green beans, trimmed

2 tablespoons olive oil

4 cloves garlic, minced

1/4 teaspoon red pepper flakes

(per serving, 1 cup):

Salt and black pepper

Calories: 100

1 tablespoon lemon juice

Fat: 8g

Protein: 2g

Wash and trim the green beans. If using fresh beans, cut them into bite-sized pieces if desired.

Bring a large pot of salted water to a boil. Add the green beans and cook for 3-4 minutes until tender-crisp. Drain and immediately transfer them to a bowl of ice water to stop the cooking process. Drain again and pat dry.

In a large skillet, heat the olive oil over medium heat. Add the minced garlic and red pepper flakes (if using) and sauté for 1-2 minutes until fragrant, being careful not to burn the garlic.

Add the drained green beans to the skillet. Sauté for 5-6 minutes, stirring occasionally, until the beans are heated through and slightly crispy.

Season with salt, black pepper, and lemon juice if using. Stir well to combine.

Transfer to a serving dish and enjoy it warm.

Sweet Potato Fries

Gluten-Free: Yes

Dairy-Free: Yes

Vegan: Yes

Prep Time: 10 minutes Cooking Time: 25 minutes Total Time: 35 minutes Serving Size: 1 cup (about 130 grams)

Calories: 150

Fat: 7g

Protein: 2g

Carbohydrates: 22g

Fiber: 4g

Sugars: 7g

2 medium sweet potatoes

1-2 tablespoons olive oil or other cooking oil of choice

1/2 teaspoon paprika

1/2 teaspoon garlic powder

1/4 teaspoon ground cumin

1/4 teaspoon black pepper

1/4 teaspoon sea salt

1/4 teaspoon cayenne pepper

Preheat your oven to 425°F (220°C). Line a baking sheet with parchment paper or lightly grease it.

Peel the sweet potatoes and cut them into thin strips (about 1/4 inch thick) to resemble fries.

In a large bowl, toss the sweet potato strips with olive oil, paprika, garlic powder, cumin, black pepper, and sea salt until evenly coated.

Spread the seasoned sweet potato strips in a single layer on the prepared baking sheet. Make sure they are not overlapping to ensure even cooking.

Bake in the preheated oven for 20-25 minutes, flipping halfway through, until the fries are golden brown and crispy.

Remove from the oven and let cool slightly before serving. Enjoy the warmth.

CHAPTER 7

VEGETARIAN AND VEGAN

Caprese-Stuffed Portobello Mushrooms

Gluten-Free: Yes

Dairy-Free: No

Vegan: No

Prep Time: 10 minutes Cooking Time: 20 minutes Total Time: 30 minutes Serving Size: 1 mushroom cap (makes 4 servings)

Calories: 150

Fat: 10g

Protein: 7g

Carbohydrates: 10g

Fiber: 2g

Sugars: 6g

- 4 large portobello mushroom caps
- 1 cup cherry tomatoes, halved
- 1 cup fresh basil leaves, chopped
- 1/2 cup mozzarella cheese, shredded
- 2 tablespoons extra virgin olive oil
- 1 tablespoon balsamic vinegar
- 1 clove garlic, minced
- Salt and black pepper

Preheat your oven to 375°F (190°C).

Clean the portobello mushroom caps with a damp paper towel. Remove the stems and scoop out the gills using a spoon.

In a mixing bowl, combine the cherry tomatoes, chopped basil, mozzarella cheese, minced garlic, olive oil, balsamic vinegar, salt, and black pepper.

Place the mushroom caps on a baking sheet lined with parchment paper. Spoon the tomato and cheese mixture into each mushroom cap, distributing it evenly.

Bake in the preheated oven for 20 minutes, or until the mushrooms are tender and the cheese is melted and bubbly.

Remove from the oven and let cool for a few minutes before serving.

Sweet Potato-Black Bean Tacos

Gluten-Free: Yes

Dairy-Free: Yes

Vegan: Yes

Prep Time: 15 minutes Cooking Time: 20 minutes Total Time: 35 minutes Serving Size: 2 tacos (about 1 cup filling per taco)

(per serving, 2 tacos):

Calories: 350

Fat: 8g

Protein: 12g

Carbohydrates: 56g

Fiber: 12g

Sugars: 10g

- 1 large sweet potato, peeled and diced
- 1 tablespoon olive oil
- 1/2 teaspoon ground cumin
- 1/2 teaspoon paprika
- 1/4 teaspoon ground turmeric
- 1/4 teaspoon garlic powder
- 1/4 teaspoon onion powder
- Salt and black pepper
- 1 can (15 oz) black beans, drained and rinsed
- 1/2 cup diced red onion
- 1/2 cup diced bell pepper (any color)
- 1/4 cup chopped fresh cilantro
- Juice of 1 lime
- 4 small corn or gluten-free tortillas
- Optional toppings: avocado slices, salsa, shredded lettuce, chopped tomatoes

Preheat the oven to 400°F (200°C). Toss the diced sweet potato with olive oil, cumin, paprika, turmeric, garlic powder, onion powder, salt, and pepper. Spread evenly on a baking sheet.

Roast in the oven for 20 minutes or until tender and lightly browned, stirring halfway through.

In a bowl, combine black beans, diced red onion, diced bell pepper, cilantro, and lime juice. Season with salt and pepper to taste.

Heat the tortillas in a dry skillet over medium heat until warm and pliable, about 30 seconds per side.

Fill each tortilla with roasted sweet potatoes and black bean mixture. Top with optional toppings if desired..

Lentil and Spinach Stew

Gluten-Free: Yes

Dairy-Free: Yes

Vegan: Yes

Prep Time: 10 minutes Cooking Time: 30 minutes Total Time: 40 minutes Serving Size: 1 cup (about 8 ounces)

(per serving, 1 cup):

Calories: 180

Fat: 5g

Protein: 9g

Carbohydrates: 27g

Fiber: 9g

Sugars: 6g

1 tablespoon olive oil

1 medium onion, diced

3 garlic cloves, minced

1 large carrot, diced

1 celery stalk, diced

1 cup dried green or brown lentils, rinsed

1 can (14.5 ounces) diced tomatoes

4 cups vegetable broth

2 cups fresh spinach, chopped

1 teaspoon ground turmeric

1/2 teaspoon ground cumin

1/2 teaspoon smoked paprika

1/4 teaspoon ground black pepper

1/4 teaspoon sea salt

1 bay leaf

Heat olive oil in a large pot over medium heat. Add the onion, garlic, carrot, and celery. Cook for about 5-7 minutes, or until the vegetables are softened.

Stir in the turmeric, cumin, paprika, black pepper, and salt. Cook for another 1-2 minutes until fragrant.

Add the lentils, diced tomatoes, vegetable broth, and bay leaf (if using). Bring to a boil.

Reduce the heat to low and let the stew simmer for about 20-25 minutes, or until the lentils are tender.

Stir in the chopped spinach and cook for an additional 5 minutes, until the spinach is wilted and the stew is heated through.

Taste and adjust seasoning if needed. Remove the bay leaf before serving.

Ladle into bowls

Vegetable Paella

Gluten-Free: Yes

Dairy-Free: Yes

Vegan: Yes

Prep Time: 15 minutes Cooking Time: 35 minutes Total Time: 50 minutes Serving Size: 1 cup (about 200g)

Calories: 250

Fat: 7g

Protein: 7g

Carbohydrates: 40g

Fiber: 7g

Sugars: 8g

1 tablespoon olive oil

1 onion, finely chopped

3 garlic cloves, minced

1 red bell pepper, chopped

1 yellow bell pepper, chopped

1 zucchini, sliced

1 cup cherry tomatoes, halved

1 cup green beans, trimmed and cut into pieces

1 cup peas (fresh or frozen)

1 1/2 cups short-grain brown rice

1/4 teaspoon saffron threads or 1/2 teaspoon turmeric as a substitute

1 teaspoon smoked paprika

1/2 teaspoon ground cumin

1/4 teaspoon ground black pepper

1/4 teaspoon cayenne pepper

3 cups vegetable broth

1 lemon, cut into wedges

Fresh parsley, chopped

Heat the olive oil in a large skillet or paella pan over medium heat. Add the onion and garlic and cook until softened, about 5 minutes.

Stir in the red and yellow bell peppers and zucchini. Cook for another 5 minutes, until vegetables begin to soften.

Add the saffron (or turmeric), smoked paprika, cumin, black pepper, and cayenne pepper (if using). Stir to coat the vegetables in the spices.

Stir in the rice, making sure it is well-coated with the spices. Pour in the vegetable broth and bring to a boil.

Reduce heat to low, cover, and simmer for about 20 minutes.

After 20 minutes, add the cherry tomatoes, green beans, and peas. Stir gently, cover, and cook for another 10 minutes, or until the rice is tender and the liquid has been absorbed.

Remove from heat and let the paella sit, covered, for 5 minutes.

Garnish with chopped parsley and serve with lemon wedges.

Mushroom Risotto

Gluten-Free: Yes

Dairy-Free: No

Vegan: Yes

Prep Time: 10 minutes Cooking Time: 30 minutes Total Time: 40 minutes Serving Size: 1 cup

Calories: 250

Fat: 8g

Protein: 5g

Carbohydrates: 40g

Fiber: 2g

Sugars: 4g

1 cup Arborio rice

1 tablespoon olive oil

1 medium onion, finely chopped

2 cloves garlic, minced

2 cups mushrooms, sliced

1/4 cup white wine

4 cups vegetable broth

1/4 cup nutritional yeast

2 tablespoons fresh parsley, chopped

Salt and pepper

Heat the vegetable broth in a saucepan and keep it warm on low heat.

In a large skillet, heat the olive oil over medium heat. Add the chopped onion and cook until translucent, about 5 minutes. Add the garlic and mushrooms and cook until the mushrooms are softened, about 5 minutes.

Stir in the Arborio rice and cook for 1-2 minutes until lightly toasted.

If using white wine, add it now and cook until the wine is mostly absorbed.

Begin adding the warm vegetable broth, one ladleful at a time, stirring frequently. Allow the liquid to be absorbed before adding more broth. Continue this process until the rice is creamy and cooked through, about 20-25 minutes.

Stir in the nutritional yeast, if using, and season with salt and pepper.

Garnish with fresh parsley.

Chickpea and Spinach Curry

Gluten-Free: Yes

Dairy-Free: Yes

Vegan: Yes

Prep Time: 10 minutes Cooking Time: 25 minutes Total Time: 35 minutes Serving Size: 1 cup (about 8 ounces)

Calories: 250

Fat: 14g

Protein: 8g

Carbohydrates: 28g

Fiber: 7g

Sugars: 6g

- 1 tablespoon olive oil
- 1 onion, finely chopped
- 3 garlic cloves, minced
- 1 tablespoon fresh ginger, minced
- 1 can (15 oz) chickpeas, drained and rinsed
- 1 can (15 oz) diced tomatoes
- 1 cup coconut milk
- 2 cups fresh spinach, chopped
- 1 tablespoon curry powder
- 1/2 teaspoon ground turmeric
- 1/2 teaspoon ground cumin
- 1/2 teaspoon ground coriander
- 1/4 teaspoon cayenne pepper
- Salt and black pepper
- Fresh cilantro

In a large skillet or saucepan, heat the olive oil over medium heat.

Add the onion and cook until translucent, about 5 minutes. Add the garlic and ginger and cook for another 1-2 minutes.

Stir in the curry powder, turmeric, cumin, coriander, and cayenne pepper (if using). Cook for 1 minute to toast the spices.

Add the chickpeas and diced tomatoes to the skillet. Stir well to combine.

Pour in the coconut milk, bring the mixture to a simmer, and cook for 10 minutes, allowing the flavors to meld and the sauce to thicken slightly.

Stir in the chopped spinach and cook for an additional 5 minutes until the spinach is wilted.

Season with salt and black pepper to taste.

Garnish with fresh cilantro if desired and serve hot.

Vegan Buddha Bowl

Gluten-Free: Yes

Dairy-Free: Yes

Vegan: Yes

Prep Time: 15 minutes **Cooking Time:** 20 minutes **Total Time:** 35 minutes **Serving Size:** 1 bowl

Calories: 500

Fat: 22g

Protein: 14g

Carbohydrates: 60g

Fiber: 12g

Sugars: 9g

For the Bowl:

1 cup cooked quinoa

1 cup roasted sweet potatoes (cubed)

1 cup steamed broccoli florets

1/2 cup shredded red cabbage

1/2 avocado, sliced

1/4 cup chickpeas (cooked or canned, rinsed)

2 tablespoons sesame seeds

For the Dressing:

2 tablespoons tahini

1 tablespoon lemon juice

1 tablespoon tamari (gluten-free soy sauce) or coconut aminos

1 teaspoon maple syrup

1 clove garlic, minced

Water, as needed to thin the dressing

Rinse quinoa under cold water. Cook according to package instructions (usually 1 part quinoa to 2 parts water, bring to a boil, then simmer for about 15 minutes). Let cool.

Preheat the oven to 400°F (200°C). Toss cubed sweet potatoes with a bit of olive oil, salt, and pepper. Spread on a baking sheet and roast for 20 minutes, or until tender.

Steam broccoli florets for about 5-7 minutes until tender but still crisp. Set aside.

In a small bowl, whisk together tahini, lemon juice, tamari or coconut aminos, maple syrup, and minced garlic. Add water a little at a time

until the dressing reaches your desired consistency.

In a large bowl, arrange cooked quinoa, roasted sweet potatoes, steamed broccoli, shredded red cabbage, avocado slices, and chickpeas. Drizzle with tahini dressing and sprinkle with sesame seeds.

Vegan Lentil Soup

Gluten-Free: Yes

Dairy-Free: Yes

Vegan: Yes

Prep Time: 10 minutes Cooking Time: 30 minutes Total Time: 40 minutes Serving Size: 1 cup

Calories: 180

Fat: 4g

Protein: 10g

Carbs: 28g

Fiber: 9g

Sugars: 6g

- 1 tablespoon olive oil
- 1 medium onion, diced
- 2 cloves garlic, minced
- 2 medium carrots, diced
- 2 celery stalks, diced
- 1 cup dried green or brown lentils, rinsed and drained
- 1 can (14.5 ounces) diced tomatoes
- 6 cups vegetable broth (ensure gluten-free if needed)
- 1 teaspoon ground cumin
- 1 teaspoon smoked paprika
- 1/2 teaspoon ground turmeric
- 1/2 teaspoon dried thyme
- 1 bay leaf
- Salt and pepper
- 2 cups spinach or kale, chopped

In a large pot, heat the olive oil over medium heat. Add the onion and garlic, and sauté until the onion is translucent, about 5 minutes.

Stir in the carrots and celery and cook for an additional 5 minutes.

Add the lentils, diced tomatoes, vegetable broth, cumin, paprika, turmeric, thyme, bay leaf, salt, and pepper. Bring to a boil.

Reduce heat and let the soup simmer for 25-30 minutes, or until the lentils and vegetables are tender.

If using spinach or kale, stir it in during the last 5 minutes of cooking.

Remove the bay leaf before serving. Adjust seasoning to taste.

CHAPTER 8

FISH AND SEAFOOD

Turmeric-Spiced Shrimp

Gluten-Free: Yes

Dairy-Free: Yes

Vegan: No

Prep Time: 10 minutes Cooking Time: 10 minutes Total Time: 20 minutes Serving Size: 2 servings (about 4-6 shrimp per serving)

Calories: 150

Fat: 8g

Protein: 18g

Carbohydrates: 2g

Fiber: 0g

Sugars: 0g

- 12 large shrimp, peeled and deveined
- 1 tablespoon olive oil
- 1 teaspoon ground turmeric
- 1/2 teaspoon ground cumin
- 1/2 teaspoon paprika
- 1/4 teaspoon ground black pepper
- 1/4 teaspoon garlic powder
- 1/4 teaspoon ground ginger
- 1/4 teaspoon salt
- 1 tablespoon lemon juice
- Fresh cilantro or parsley

In a medium bowl, combine the olive oil, turmeric, cumin, paprika, black pepper, garlic powder, ginger, salt, and lemon juice. Add the shrimp and toss to coat evenly. Let it marinate for at least 10 minutes.

Heat a large skillet over medium heat.

Add the marinated shrimp to the hot skillet. Cook for 2-3 minutes on each side, or until the shrimp are opaque and cooked through.

Transfer the shrimp to a plate and garnish with fresh cilantro or parsley, if desired..

Mackerel and Olive Relish

Gluten-Free: Yes

Dairy-Free: Yes

Vegan: No

Prep Time: 10 minutes Cooking Time: 10 minutes Total Time: 20 minutes Serving Size: 2 servings

Calories: 350

Fat: 25g

Protein: 25g

Carbohydrates: 8g

Fiber: 3g

Sugars: 4g

For the Mackerel:

2 mackerel filets

1 tablespoon olive oil

Salt and pepper

1 lemon (cut in half, one half juiced, the other half cut into wedges for serving)

For the Tomato and Olive Relish:

1 cup cherry tomatoes, quartered

1/4 cup Kalamata olives, pitted and sliced

1 tablespoon capers, drained

1 small red onion, finely chopped

2 tablespoons fresh parsley, chopped

1 tablespoon extra-virgin olive oil

1 tablespoon balsamic vinegar

Salt and pepper

Prepare the Mackerel:

Season the mackerel filets with salt, pepper, and lemon juice.

Heat the olive oil in a large skillet over medium-high heat.

Add the mackerel filets, skin-side down, and cook for 3-4 minutes until the skin is crispy.

Flip the filets and cook for another 2-3 minutes until the fish is cooked through.

Make the Tomato and Olive Relish:

In a medium bowl, combine the cherry tomatoes, olives, capers, red onion, parsley, olive oil, and balsamic vinegar.

Season the relish with salt and pepper to taste and toss well.

Serve:

Plate the mackerel filets and spoon the tomato and olive relish over the top.

Serve with lemon wedges on the side.

Sardine Salad

Gluten-Free: Yes

Dairy-Free: Yes

Vegan: No

Prep Time: 10 minutes **Serving Size:** 1 salad

1 can (3.75 oz) sardines packed in olive oil, drained

1 cup mixed greens

1/4 cup cherry tomatoes, halved

1/4 cucumber, sliced

1/4 red onion, thinly sliced

1 tablespoon capers, drained

1 tablespoon fresh lemon juice

1 tablespoon extra-virgin olive oil

1/2 avocado, sliced

Salt and pepper

Optional: Fresh herbs like parsley or dill for garnish

Calories: 350

Fat: 28g

Protein: 18g

Carbohydrates: 8g

Fiber: 5g

Sugars: 2g

Place the mixed greens in a large bowl or on a plate.

Top the greens with cherry tomatoes, cucumber, red onion, and capers.

Gently place the sardines on top of the salad.

Drizzle the salad with lemon juice and olive oil. Season with salt and pepper to taste.

Arrange the avocado slices around the salad

Garnish with fresh herbs if desired..

Tuna and White Bean Salad

Gluten-Free: Yes

Dairy-Free: Yes

Vegan: No

Prep Time: 10 minutes **Serving Size:** 2 servings

Calories: 320

Fat: 14g

Protein: 27g

Carbohydrates: 24g

Fiber: 8g

Sugars: 2g

- 1 can (5 oz) tuna packed in water, drained
- 1 can (15 oz) white beans, drained and rinsed
- 1/4 cup red onion, finely chopped
- 1/4 cup fresh parsley, chopped
- 2 tablespoons extra virgin olive oil
- 1 tablespoon lemon juice (freshly squeezed)
- 1 teaspoon Dijon mustard
- Salt and pepper to taste
- Optional: 1/2 cup cherry tomatoes, halved; 1/4 cup cucumber, diced

Drain and rinse the white beans. Drain the tuna. Chop the red onion, parsley, and any optional vegetables you wish to add.

In a large bowl, combine the tuna, white beans, red onion, and parsley. Add the cherry tomatoes and cucumber if using.

In a small bowl, whisk together the olive oil, lemon juice, Dijon mustard, salt, and pepper.

Pour the dressing over the tuna and bean mixture. Toss gently until everything is well coated.

Divide the salad into two portions and serve immediately or refrigerate for later..

Garlic-Lemon Scallops

Gluten-Free: Yes

Dairy-Free: Yes

Vegan: No

Prep Time: 10 minutes Cooking Time: 10 minutes Total Time: 20 minutes Serving Size: 2 servings

Calories: 250

Fat: 14g

Protein: 25g

Carbohydrates: 6g

Fiber: 1g

Sugars: 1g

1 lb large sea scallops, cleaned and patted dry

2 tablespoons olive oil or avocado oil

3 garlic cloves, minced

Juice and zest of 1 lemon

1 tablespoon fresh parsley, chopped

Salt and pepper

Lemon wedges

Pat the scallops dry with a paper towel to ensure a good sear. Season both sides with salt and pepper.

Heat the olive oil in a large skillet over medium-high heat. Once the oil is hot, add the scallops in a single layer. Sear for about 2-3 minutes on each side until they develop a golden-brown crust. Remove the scallops from the pan and set aside.

In the same pan, reduce the heat to medium and add the minced garlic. Sauté for 1 minute, stirring constantly, until fragrant.

Add the lemon juice and zest to the pan, stirring to combine with the garlic.

Place the scallops back into the pan, tossing them in the garlic-lemon

sauce. Cook for another minute to heat through.

Transfer the scallops to a serving plate, drizzle with any remaining sauce from the pan, and sprinkle with fresh parsley. Serve with lemon wedges on the side.

Herring with Beet Salad

Gluten-Free: Yes

Dairy-Free: Yes

Vegan: No

Prep Time: 15 minutes Cooking Time: 30 minutes Total Time: 45 minutes Serving Size: 1 plate (about 1 cup salad and 1 herring filet)

Calories: 300

Fat: 15g

Protein: 15g

Carbs: 25g

Fiber: 5g

Sugars: 10g

For the Salad:

2 medium beets, cooked and diced

1 small red onion, finely chopped

1 apple, diced

1 tablespoon fresh dill, chopped

1 tablespoon apple cider vinegar

2 tablespoons olive oil

Salt and pepper

For the Herring:

1-2 herring filets (pickled or smoked)

Lemon wedges

Fresh dill

If using raw beets, boil or roast them until tender, about 30 minutes. Let them cool, then peel and dice.

In a large bowl, combine the diced beets, chopped red onion, and diced apple (if using). Add the fresh dill, apple cider vinegar, and olive oil. Toss well to combine. Season with salt and pepper to taste.

Place the herring filets on a plate. Squeeze a little lemon juice over the top and garnish with fresh dill, if desired.

Plate the beet salad alongside the herring filets..

Blackened Catfish

Gluten-Free: Yes

Dairy-Free: Yes

Prep Time: 10 minutes Cooking Time: 10 minutes Total Time: 20 minutes Serving Size: 1 filet (about 6 ounces)

Vegan: No

2 catfish filets (about 6 ounces each)

2 tablespoons olive oil or avocado oil

1 tablespoon smoked paprika

Calories: 290

1 teaspoon garlic powder

Fat: 18g

1 teaspoon onion powder

Protein: 28g

1 teaspoon dried thyme

Carbohydrates: 2g

1 teaspoon dried oregano

Fiber: 1g

1/2 teaspoon cayenne pepper

Sugars: 0g

1/2 teaspoon ground black pepper

1/2 teaspoon sea salt

Lemon wedges

In a small bowl, mix together the smoked paprika, garlic powder, onion powder, thyme, oregano, cayenne pepper, black pepper, and sea salt.

Pat the catfish filets dry with a paper towel. Generously coat both sides of the filets with the spice mixture, pressing it in so it adheres well.

Heat the olive oil or avocado oil in a large skillet over medium-high heat until it's hot but not smoking.

Carefully place the seasoned catfish filets in the skillet. Cook for about 4-5 minutes on each side, or until the fish is cooked through and the outside is blackened and crispy.

Remove the filets from the skillet and serve immediately with lemon wedges on the side..

Seaweed and Tuna Wrap

Gluten-Free: Yes

Dairy-Free: Yes

Vegan: No

Prep Time: 10 minutes Serving Size: 1 wrap

Calories: 300

Fat: 18g

Protein: 24g

Carbohydrates: 9g

Fiber: 4g

Sugars: 2g

1 sheet of nori (seaweed)

1 can (5 oz) tuna, drained

1 tablespoon mayonnaise (use avocado or olive oil-based for a healthier option)

1/4 avocado, sliced

1/4 cup shredded carrots

1/4 cup cucumber, julienned

1/4 cup mixed greens or spinach

1 teaspoon sesame seeds

A splash of tamari or coconut aminos

A few drops of lemon juice

In a bowl, mix the drained tuna with mayonnaise, sesame seeds (if using), and a few drops of lemon juice. Stir until well combined.

Lay the nori sheet on a flat surface. Spread the tuna mixture evenly over the sheet, leaving a small border around the edges.

Layer the avocado slices, shredded carrots, cucumber, and mixed greens on top of the tuna.

Carefully roll the nori sheet tightly around the fillings, similar to rolling sushi. If needed, wet the edge of the nori sheet slightly to help it stick.

Slice the wrap in half or into bite-sized pieces and serve with a splash of tamari or coconut aminos on the side..

Lemon-Dill Baked Trout

Gluten-Free: Yes

Dairy-Free: Yes

Vegan: No

Prep Time: 10 minutes Cooking Time: 20 minutes Total Time: 30 minutes Serving Size: 1 trout filet (about 6 ounces)

1 trout filet (about 6 ounces)

1 tablespoon fresh dill, chopped

1 lemon, sliced into thin rounds

1 tablespoon olive oil

Calories: 250

1 garlic clove, minced

Fat: 15g

Salt and pepper

Protein: 23g

A pinch of paprika for extra flavor

Carbohydrates: 2g

Fiber: 1g

Preheat your oven to 375°F (190°C).

Sugars: 0g

Place the trout filet on a baking sheet lined with parchment paper or lightly greased.

Drizzle the olive oil over the trout filet. Sprinkle it with minced garlic, chopped dill, salt, and pepper. Lay the lemon slices on top of the filet.

Place the baking sheet in the preheated oven and bake for 15-20 minutes, or until the trout is cooked through and flakes easily with a fork.

Remove from the oven and transfer the filet to a plate. Serve with additional lemon slices if desired.

Miso-Glazed Salmon

Gluten-Free: No

Dairy-Free: Yes

Vegan: No

Prep Time: 10 minutes Cooking Time: 15 minutes Total Time: 25 minutes Serving Size: 1 filet (about 6 ounces)

Calories: 350

Fat: 20g

Protein: 30g

Carbohydrates: 10g

Fiber: 0g

Sugars: 7g

- 2 tablespoons miso paste (ensure it's gluten-free if needed)
- 1 tablespoon rice vinegar
- 1 tablespoon honey or maple syrup
- 1 tablespoon soy sauce (use tamari for gluten-free)
- 1 teaspoon sesame oil
- 1 teaspoon grated fresh ginger
- 2 salmon filets (about 6 ounces each)
- 1 teaspoon sesame seeds
- 2 green onions, thinly sliced

Preheat your oven to 400°F (200°C).

In a small bowl, whisk together the miso paste, rice vinegar, honey or maple syrup, soy sauce (or tamari), sesame oil, and grated ginger until smooth.

Place the salmon filets on a lined baking sheet. Brush the miso glaze generously over the top of each filet.

Bake the salmon in the preheated oven for 12-15 minutes, or until the fish flakes easily with a fork.

Remove the salmon from the oven and sprinkle with sesame seeds and sliced green onions, if using. Serve immediately.

CHAPTER 9

POULTRY AND MEATS

Turmeric Chicken

Gluten-Free: Yes

Dairy-Free: Yes

Vegan: No

Prep Time: 15 minutes Cooking Time: 25 minutes Total Time: 40 minutes Serving Size: 1 serving (about 4 ounces of chicken)

(per serving, based on 4 servings total):

Calories: 250

Fat: 18g

Protein: 21g

Carbs: 2g

Fiber: 0.5g

Sugars: 0g

- 4 boneless, skinless chicken thighs (about 1 pound)
- 2 tablespoons olive oil
- 2 teaspoons ground turmeric
- 1 teaspoon ground cumin
- 1 teaspoon paprika
- 1/2 teaspoon ground black pepper
- 1/2 teaspoon garlic powder
- 1/2 teaspoon onion powder
- 1/2 teaspoon salt or to taste
- 1 tablespoon lemon juice
- 1 tablespoon chopped fresh cilantro

Preheat your oven to 375°F (190°C).

Pat the chicken thighs dry with paper towels.

In a small bowl, mix the turmeric, cumin, paprika, black pepper, garlic powder, onion powder, and salt. Rub this spice mixture all over the chicken thighs.

Heat olive oil in an oven-proof skillet over medium-high heat. Add the chicken thighs and seat for 3-4 minutes on each side, until golden brown.

Transfer the skillet to the preheated oven and bake for 20-25 minutes, or until the chicken is fully cooked and reaches an internal temperature of 165°F (74°C).

Remove from the oven, drizzle with lemon juice, and garnish with

chopped cilantro if desired.

Serve warm with your choice of side dishes.

Ginger-Garlic Chicken Stir-Fry

Gluten-Free: Yes

Dairy-Free: Yes

Vegan: No

Prep Time: 15 minutes Cooking Time: 10 minutes Total Time: 25 minutes Serving Size: 1 cup

Calories: 250

Fat: 10g

Protein: 30g

Carbohydrates: 15g

Fiber: 4g

Sugars: 6g

- 1 lb (450g) chicken breast, thinly sliced
- 1 tablespoon olive oil
- 2 cloves garlic, minced
- 1 tablespoon fresh ginger, minced
- 1 red bell pepper, sliced
- 1 cup broccoli florets
- 1 medium carrot, julienned
- 2 tablespoons coconut aminos or gluten-free soy sauce
- 1 tablespoon rice vinegar
- 1 teaspoon sesame oil
- 1 tablespoon chopped fresh cilantro
- Salt and pepper

Slice the chicken breast and vegetables. Mince the garlic and ginger.

In a large skillet or wok, heat the olive oil over medium-high heat.

Add the sliced chicken to the skillet and cook for 5-7 minutes, or until the chicken is no longer pink and starts to brown.

Add the minced garlic and ginger to the skillet. Stir-fry for 1 minute until fragrant.

Add the bell pepper, broccoli, and carrot to the skillet. Stir-fry for another 5 minutes, or until the vegetables are tender-crisp.

Stir in the coconut aminos and rice vinegar. Cook for an additional 1-2 minutes, ensuring everything is well-coated and heated through.

Drizzle with sesame oil if using, and season with salt and pepper to taste.

Garnish with chopped cilantro if desired, and serve warm..

Lemon-Herb Roasted Chicken

Gluten-Free: Yes

Dairy-Free: Yes

Paleo: Yes

Whole30: Yes

Prep Time: 15 minutes **Cooking Time:** 1 hour 15 minutes **Total Time:** 1 hour 30 minutes **Serving Size:** 1 chicken breast (about 4 ounces)

(per serving, based on 4 servings):

Calories: 300

Fat: 16g

Protein: 35g

Carbohydrates: 2g

Fiber: 0g

Sugars: 1g

- 1 whole chicken (about 4 pounds)
- 2 tablespoons olive oil
- 1 lemon, cut into wedges
- 4 cloves garlic, minced
- 2 tablespoons fresh rosemary, chopped or 2 teaspoons dried rosemary
- 2 tablespoons fresh thyme, chopped or 2 teaspoons dried thyme
- 1 teaspoon paprika
- 1 teaspoon ground black pepper
- 1 teaspoon sea salt
- 1 onion, quartered
- 1 cup low-sodium chicken broth

Preheat your oven to 425°F (220°C).

Pat the chicken dry with paper towels. Rub the outside of the chicken with olive oil.

Sprinkle garlic, rosemary, thyme, paprika, black pepper, and sea salt all over the chicken, including inside the cavity. Place the lemon wedges and quartered onion inside the cavity.

Place the chicken on a rack in a roasting pan. Roast in the preheated oven for about 1 hour to 1 hour and 15 minutes, or until the internal temperature reaches 165°F (74°C) and the skin is golden brown and crispy. Baste occasionally with chicken broth if using.

Remove the chicken from the oven and let it rest for about 10-15 minutes before carving.

Spicy Chicken Lettuce Wraps

Gluten-Free: Yes

Dairy-Free: Yes

Vegan: No

Prep Time: 15 minutes Cooking Time: 10 minutes Total Time: 25 minutes Serving Size: 4 wraps (about 1 cup of filling per wrap)

(per serving, 4 wraps):

Calories:300

Fat: 18g

Protein: 25g

Carbohydrates: 12g

Fiber: 3g

Sugars: 6g

1 lb ground chicken

1 tablespoon olive oil

1 small onion, finely chopped

2 cloves garlic, minced

1 tablespoon fresh ginger, minced

1 red bell pepper, finely chopped

1 cup shredded carrots

2 tablespoons coconut aminos or gluten-free soy sauce alternative

1 tablespoon chili paste or hot sauce

1 teaspoon ground cumin

1 teaspoon paprika

Salt and pepper to taste

12 large lettuce leaves

1/4 cup chopped fresh cilantro

Lime wedges

In a large skillet, heat the olive oil over medium heat.

Add the onion, garlic, and ginger to the skillet. Sauté for about 3 minutes until fragrant and translucent.

Add the ground chicken to the skillet. Cook, breaking it up with a spoon, until browned and cooked through, about 5-7 minutes.

Stir in the red bell pepper and shredded carrots. Cook for an additional 2-3 minutes until vegetables are tender.

Add the coconut aminos, chili paste or hot sauce, ground cumin, paprika, salt, and pepper. Mix well and cook for another 2 minutes, allowing the flavors to combine.

Wash and dry the lettuce leaves. Arrange them on a serving platter.

Spoon the spicy chicken mixture into the center of each lettuce leaf.

Garnish with chopped cilantro and serve with lime wedges on the side, if desired.

Chicken and Sweet Potato Stew

Gluten-Free: Yes

Dairy-Free: Yes

Paleo: Yes

Whole30: Yes

Prep Time: 15 minutes Cooking Time: 45 minutes Total Time: 1 hour
Serving Size: 1 cup (about 8 ounces)

(per serving, 1 cup):

Calories: 250

Fat: 10g

Protein: 23g

Carbohydrates: 24g

Fiber: 5g

Sugars: 6g

- 1 lb (450g) boneless, skinless chicken thighs, cut into bite-sized pieces
- 2 medium sweet potatoes, peeled and diced
- 1 large carrot, peeled and sliced
- 1 onion, chopped
- 3 cloves garlic, minced
- 1 tablespoon olive oil
- 1 teaspoon ground turmeric
- 1 teaspoon ground cumin
- 1/2 teaspoon ground paprika
- 1/2 teaspoon dried thyme
- 1/2 teaspoon dried rosemary
- 4 cups low-sodium chicken broth
- 1 cup chopped kale or spinach
- Salt and pepper

Peel and dice the sweet potatoes and carrot. Chop the onion and mince the garlic.

In a large pot or Dutch oven, heat the olive oil over medium heat. Add the chopped onion and cook until translucent, about 5 minutes.

Add the chicken pieces and cook until lightly browned on all sides, about 5-7 minutes.

Stir in the minced garlic, turmeric, cumin, paprika, thyme, and rosemary. Cook for 1 minute until fragrant.

Add the diced sweet potatoes, sliced carrot, and chicken broth. Stir to combine.

Bring the stew to a boil, then reduce the heat to low. Cover and simmer for 30-35 minutes, or until the sweet potatoes and carrots are tender and the chicken is cooked through.

If using, stir in the chopped kale or spinach and cook for an additional 5 minutes until wilted.

Season with salt and pepper to taste.

Rosemary Garlic Lamb Chops

Gluten-Free: Yes

Dairy-Free: Yes

Paleo: Yes

Keto: Yes

Prep Time: 10 minutes Cooking Time: 15 minutes Total Time: 25 minutes Serving Size: 2 lamb chops

4 lamb chops about 1 inch thick

2 tablespoons olive oil

3 cloves garlic, minced

2 tablespoons fresh rosemary, chopped or 2 teaspoons dried rosemary

1 teaspoon salt

1/2 teaspoon black pepper

1/2 teaspoon lemon zest

per serving, 2 lamb chops):

Calories: 350

Fat: 24g

Protein: 30g

Carbohydrates: 0g

Fiber: 0g

Sugars: 0g

In a small bowl, combine olive oil, minced garlic, rosemary, salt, pepper, and lemon zest (if using). Rub this mixture all over the lamb chops.

Allow the lamb chops to marinate for at least 10 minutes. For more intense flavor, you can marinate them for up to 1 hour in the refrigerator.

Heat a large skillet or grill pan over medium-high heat.

Add the lamb chops to the hot pan. Cook for about 4-5 minutes per side for medium-rare, or longer if desired.

Remove the lamb chops from the pan and let them rest for 5 minutes before serving.

Ginger-Turmeric Beef Stir-Fry

Gluten-Free: Yes

Dairy-Free: Yes

Vegan: No

Prep Time: 15 minutes Cooking Time: 10 minutes Total Time: 25 minutes Serving Size: 1 cup (about 1 serving)

Calories: 350

Fat: 20g

Protein: 30g

Carbohydrates: 15g

Fiber: 4g

Sugars: 7g

- 1 pound (450g) beef sirloin, thinly sliced
- 1 tablespoon coconut oil
- 1 tablespoon fresh ginger, minced
- 1 tablespoon fresh turmeric, minced or 1 teaspoon ground turmeric
- 2 cups bell peppers, sliced (red and yellow)
- 1 cup broccoli florets
- 1 medium carrot, sliced
- 1 tablespoon tamari (gluten-free soy sauce) or coconut aminos
- 1 tablespoon lime juice
- 1 tablespoon sesame seeds
- Salt and pepper

Slice the beef and vegetables. Mince the ginger and turmeric (or use ground turmeric).

In a large skillet or wok, heat the coconut oil over medium-high heat.

Add the sliced beef to the skillet and stir-fry for about 3-4 minutes until browned and cooked through. Remove beef from the skillet and set aside.

In the same skillet, add the minced ginger and turmeric. Stir-fry for about 1 minute until fragrant.

Add the bell peppers, broccoli, and carrots to the skillet. Stir-fry for about 5 minutes until vegetables are tender-crisp.

Return the cooked beef to the skillet. Add tamari or coconut aminos and lime juice. Stir to combine and cook for an additional 2 minutes.

Season with salt and pepper to taste. Garnish with sesame seeds if desired.

Serve the stir-fry hot over steamed rice or cauliflower rice.

Herb-Roasted Pork Tenderloin

Gluten-Free: Yes

Dairy-Free: Yes

Paleo: Yes

Prep Time: 10 minutes Cooking Time: 25-30 minutes Total Time: 40 minutes Serving Size: 1 slice (about 4 ounces)

Calories: 200

Fat: 10g

Protein: 28g

Carbohydrates: 1g

Fiber: 0g

Sugars: 0g

1 pound pork tenderloin

2 tablespoons olive oil

2 cloves garlic, minced

1 tablespoon fresh rosemary, chopped or 1 teaspoon dried

1 tablespoon fresh thyme, chopped or 1 teaspoon dried

1 teaspoon dried oregano

1/2 teaspoon paprika

Salt and pepper

Preheat your oven to 400°F (200°C).

Pat the pork tenderloin dry with paper towels. This helps with browning.

In a small bowl, mix together the olive oil, garlic, rosemary, thyme, oregano, paprika, salt, and pepper. Rub this mixture all over the pork tenderloin.

Heat a large ovenproof skillet over medium-high heat. Sear the pork tenderloin for about 2-3 minutes on each side until browned.

Transfer the skillet to the preheated oven and roast the pork tenderloin for 20-25 minutes, or until the internal temperature reaches 145°F (63°C).

Remove the pork from the oven and let it rest for 5-10 minutes before slicing. This helps the juices redistribute.

Slice the pork tenderloin and serve warm.

Spiced Turkey Meatballs

Calories per Serving: 200

Fat: 4g

Protein: 6g

Carbs: 34g

Prep Time: 15 minutes Cooking Time: 25 minutes Total Time: 40 minutes Serving Size: 4 meatballs (about 1.5 inches in diameter)

- 1 lb ground turkey
- 1/2 cup finely chopped onion
- 2 cloves garlic, minced
- 1/4 cup fresh parsley, chopped
- 1/4 cup almond flour
- 1 large egg
- 1 teaspoon ground cumin
- 1/2 teaspoon ground paprika
- 1/2 teaspoon ground turmeric
- 1/4 teaspoon ground black pepper
- 1/4 teaspoon ground cinnamon
- 1/2 teaspoon salt
- 1 tablespoon olive oil

(per serving of 4 meatballs):

Calories: 240

Fat: 14g

Protein: 22g

Carbohydrates: 6g

Fiber: 2g

Sugars: 1g

Preheat your oven to 400°F (200°C). Line a baking sheet with parchment paper or lightly grease it.

In a large bowl, combine the ground turkey, chopped onion, minced garlic, parsley, almond flour, egg, cumin, paprika, turmeric, black pepper, cinnamon, and salt. Mix until well combined but don't overmix.

Shape the mixture into meatballs, about 1.5 inches in diameter, and place them on the prepared baking sheet.

Drizzle the meatballs with olive oil. Bake for 20-25 minutes, or until the meatballs are cooked through and have an internal temperature of 165°F (74°C).

Let the meatballs rest for a few minutes before serving.

Beef and Vegetable Kebabs

Gluten-Free: Yes

Dairy-Free: Yes

Vegan: No

Prep Time: 15 minutes Cooking Time: 10-15 minutes Total Time: 1 hour 30 minutes Serving Size: 2 kebabs (1/2 pound of beef and vegetables)

(per serving, 2 kebabs):

Calories: 350

Fat: 20g

Protein: 30g

Carbohydrates: 15g

Fiber: 4g

Sugars: 8g

1 pound beef sirloin or tenderloin, cut into 1-inch cubes

1 red bell pepper, cut into chunks

1 green bell pepper, cut into chunks

1 zucchini, sliced into rounds

1 red onion, cut into chunks

2 tablespoons olive oil

2 tablespoons balsamic vinegar

1 tablespoon lemon juice

2 cloves garlic, minced

1 teaspoon dried oregano

1 teaspoon dried thyme

1 teaspoon paprika

1/2 teaspoon ground black pepper

1/2 teaspoon salt

In a bowl, mix olive oil, balsamic vinegar, lemon juice, garlic, oregano, thyme, paprika, black pepper, and salt.

Add beef cubes to the marinade and toss to coat. Cover and refrigerate for at least 1 hour (or overnight for more flavor).

Preheat the grill or grill pan to medium-high heat.

Thread the marinated beef, bell peppers, zucchini, and onion onto skewers, alternating between beef and vegetables.

Grill the kebabs for 10-15 minutes, turning occasionally, until the beef is cooked to your desired level of doneness and vegetables are

tender.

Remove from the grill and let rest for a few minutes before serving.

CHAPTER 10

SOUPS AND STEWS

Turmeric Chicken Soup

Gluten-Free: Yes

Dairy-Free: Yes

Vegan: No

Prep Time: 15 minutes Cooking Time: 30 minutes Total Time: 45 minutes Serving Size: 1 bowl (about 2 cups)

Calories: 300

Fat: 20g

Protein: 20g

Carbohydrates: 15g

Fiber: 4g

Sugars: 5g

- 1 lb (about 450g) boneless, skinless chicken thighs or breasts, cut into bite-sized pieces
- 1 tablespoon olive oil
- 1 large onion, diced
- 3 cloves garlic, minced
- 1 tablespoon fresh ginger, grated
- 1 tablespoon ground turmeric
- 1 teaspoon ground cumin
- 1 teaspoon ground coriander
- 4 cups chicken broth (gluten-free)
- 1 can (14 oz) coconut milk
- 2 large carrots, sliced
- 2 celery stalks, sliced
- 1 zucchini, diced
- -1 cup baby spinach
- Juice of 1 lemon
- Salt and pepper
- Fresh cilantro or parsley

In a large pot, heat the olive oil over medium heat. Add the diced onion and sauté until softened, about 5 minutes. Add the garlic and ginger, and sauté for another minute until fragrant.

Add the chicken pieces to the pot and cook until browned on all sides, about 5-7 minutes.

Stir in the turmeric, cumin, and coriander, cooking for another minute to release the spices' aromas.

Pour in the chicken broth and coconut milk (if using). Add the carrots, celery, and zucchini. Bring the soup to a boil, then reduce the heat and let it simmer for 20 minutes, until the vegetables are tender and the chicken is cooked through.

Stir in the baby spinach and lemon juice, and season with salt and pepper to taste. Cook for another 2-3 minutes, until the spinach is wilted.

Ladle the soup into bowls and garnish with fresh cilantro or parsley.

Miso Soup with Tofu

Gluten-Free: Yes

Dairy-Free: Yes

Vegan: Yes

Prep Time: 10 minutes Cooking Time: 10 minutes Total Time: 20 minutes Serving Size: 1 bowl (about 12 ounces)

4 cups water or vegetable broth

3 tablespoons miso paste (ensure it's gluten-free if necessary)

1/2 cup firm tofu, cubed

1/2 cup chopped green onions (scallions)

1/2 cup sliced shiitake mushrooms

1/4 cup wakame seaweed, rehydrated

1 tablespoon tamari or gluten-free soy sauce

Calories: 90

Fat: 3g

Protein: 7g

Carbohydrates: 8g

Fiber: 2g

Sugars: 1g

If using dried wakame seaweed, soak it in water for 5 minutes until rehydrated, then drain and set aside.

In a medium-sized pot, bring the water or vegetable broth to a gentle simmer over medium heat.

Add the tofu, green onions, shiitake mushrooms, and rehydrated wakame seaweed to the pot. Simmer for about 5 minutes until the mushrooms are tender and the tofu is heated through.

Reduce the heat to low. Place the miso paste in a small bowl, add a ladle of hot broth, and whisk until smooth. Add the diluted miso back into the soup and stir well. Do not boil the soup after adding the miso, as this can destroy its beneficial probiotics.

Add tamari or gluten-free soy sauce if desired for extra flavor. Adjust to taste.

Ladle the soup into bowls and serve warm.

Quinoa Vegetable Soup

Gluten-Free: Yes

Dairy-Free: Yes

Vegan: Yes

Prep Time: 10 minutes **Cooking Time:** 25 minutes **Total Time:** 35 minutes **Serving Size:** 1 bowl (about 1 1/2 cups)

Calories: 210

Fat: 5g

Protein: 7g

Carbohydrates: 35g

Fiber: 7g

Sugars: 7g

- 1/2 cup quinoa, rinsed
- 1 tablespoon olive oil
- 1 onion, diced
- 2 carrots, diced
- 2 celery stalks, diced
- 3 garlic cloves, minced
- 1 zucchini, diced
- 1 red bell pepper, diced
- 1 can (14.5 ounces) diced tomatoes
- 6 cups vegetable broth
- 1 teaspoon ground turmeric
- 1 teaspoon ground cumin
- 1/2 teaspoon ground coriander
- 1/2 teaspoon smoked paprika
- 1/2 teaspoon dried thyme
- Salt and pepper to taste
- 2 cups kale or spinach, chopped
- 1/4 cup fresh parsley, chopped
- 1 tablespoon lemon juice

In a medium saucepan, bring 1 cup of water to a boil. Add the quinoa, reduce the heat to low, cover, and simmer for about 15 minutes until the quinoa is cooked and the water is absorbed. Set aside.

In a large pot, heat the olive oil over medium heat. Add the onion, carrots, celery, and garlic. Sauté for 5-7 minutes until the vegetables are softened.

Stir in the zucchini, red bell pepper, and diced tomatoes. Cook for another 3 minutes.

Add the turmeric, cumin, coriander, smoked paprika, thyme, salt, and pepper. Pour in the vegetable broth, stir well, and bring the soup to a boil.

Reduce the heat and let the soup simmer for 15 minutes.

Stir in the cooked quinoa and chopped kale or spinach. Simmer for another 5 minutes until the greens are wilted.

Stir in the lemon juice if using. Ladle the soup into bowls, garnish with fresh parsley, and serve warm.

Cabbage and Kale Soup

Gluten-Free: Yes

Dairy-Free: Yes

Vegan: Yes

Prep Time: 10 minutes Cooking Time: 30 minutes Total Time: 40 minutes Serving Size: 1 bowl (about 2 cups)

Calories: 120

Fat: 4g

Protein: 4g

Carbohydrates: 18g

Fiber: 6g

Sugars: 8g

- 1 tablespoon olive oil
- 1 medium onion, diced
- 2 garlic cloves, minced
- 4 cups green cabbage, chopped
- 2 cups kale, chopped (stems removed)
- 2 carrots, sliced
- 1 celery stalk, sliced
- 1 can (14.5 oz) diced tomatoes (no salt added)
- 6 cups vegetable broth (low-sodium)
- 1 teaspoon turmeric
- 1/2 teaspoon ground cumin
- 1/2 teaspoon ground black pepper
- 1/2 teaspoon paprika
- Salt to taste
- Juice of 1/2 lemon

Heat the olive oil in a large pot over medium heat. Add the diced onion and garlic, and sauté until the onion becomes translucent, about 5 minutes.

Stir in the chopped cabbage, kale, carrots, and celery. Cook for another 5 minutes, stirring occasionally.

Add the diced tomatoes, vegetable broth, turmeric, cumin, black pepper, and paprika. Stir well to combine.

Bring the soup to a boil, then reduce the heat to low and let it simmer for 20-25 minutes, or until the vegetables are tender.

Taste and adjust the seasoning with salt if needed. Stir in the lemon juice if using, and serve the soup hot.

Turkish Red Lentil Soup

Gluten-Free: Yes

Dairy-Free: Yes

Vegan: Yes

Prep Time: 10 minutes Cooking Time: 30 minutes Total Time: 40 minutes Serving Size: 1 bowl (about 1 1/2 cups)

Calories: 180

Fat: 4g

Protein: 9g

Carbohydrates: 28g

Fiber: 7g

Sugars: 4g

- 1 cup red lentils, rinsed
- 1 medium onion, finely chopped
- 1 carrot, peeled and diced
- 2 cloves garlic, minced
- 1 tablespoon olive oil
- 1 tablespoon tomato paste
- 1 teaspoon ground cumin
- 1/2 teaspoon ground paprika or smoked paprika
- 1/4 teaspoon ground turmeric
- 1/4 teaspoon ground black pepper
- 4 cups vegetable broth or water
- 1 teaspoon salt or to taste
- 1 lemon, cut into wedges
- Fresh parsley, chopped

In a large pot, heat the olive oil over medium heat. Add the chopped onion, carrot, and garlic. Sauté for 5 minutes, or until the onion becomes translucent and the vegetables are softened.

Stir in the tomato paste, cumin, paprika, turmeric, and black pepper. Cook for an additional 2 minutes, allowing the spices to become fragrant.

Add the rinsed red lentils and vegetable broth (or water) to the pot. Stir to combine.

Bring the mixture to a boil, then reduce the heat to low. Cover and let it simmer for about 20-25 minutes, or until the lentils are soft and the soup has thickened.

For a smoother texture, use an immersion blender to blend the soup until creamy. You can also leave it chunky if you prefer.

Taste and adjust the seasoning with salt if necessary.

Ladle the soup into bowls and serve with lemon wedges for squeezing over the top. Garnish with fresh parsley if desired.

Mushroom Barley Soup

Gluten-Free: No

Dairy-Free: Yes

Vegan: Yes

Prep Time: 15 minutes Cooking Time: 45 minutes Total Time: 1 hour Serving Size: 1 bowl (about 1 1/2 cups)

Calories: 250

Fat: 5g

Protein: 7g

Carbohydrates: 45g

Fiber: 8g

Sugars: 4g

- 1 tablespoon olive oil
- 1 medium onion, diced
- 2 cloves garlic, minced
- 2 carrots, diced
- 2 celery stalks, diced
- 8 ounces mushrooms, sliced
- 1 cup pearl barley
- 6 cups vegetable broth
- 1 teaspoon dried thyme
- 1 bay leaf
- Salt and pepper
- 1 tablespoon fresh parsley, chopped

Heat olive oil in a large pot over medium heat. Add the onion, garlic, carrots, and celery. Sauté for about 5 minutes until the vegetables begin to soften.

Add the sliced mushrooms to the pot and cook for another 5 minutes until they release their moisture and begin to brown.

Stir in the pearl barley, vegetable broth, dried thyme, and bay leaf. Bring the mixture to a boil.

Reduce the heat to low, cover, and simmer for about 45 minutes, or until the barley is tender and the soup has thickened. Stir occasionally.

Remove the bay leaf, then season the soup with salt and pepper to taste.

Ladle the soup into bowls and garnish with fresh parsley if desired.

Serve hot.

Spicy Chickpea Soup

Gluten-Free: Yes

Dairy-Free: Yes

Vegan: Yes

Prep Time: 10 minutes **Cooking Time:** 30 minutes **Total Time:** 40 minutes **Serving Size:** 1 bowl (about 1.5 cups)

Calories: 250

Fat: 6g

Protein: 8g

Carbohydrates: 40g

Fiber: 10g

Sugars: 8g

- 1 tablespoon olive oil
- 1 small onion, diced
- 2 cloves garlic, minced
- 1 teaspoon ground cumin
- 1 teaspoon ground coriander
- 1/2 teaspoon ground turmeric
- 1/4 teaspoon cayenne pepper (adjust to taste)
- 1/4 teaspoon smoked paprika
- 1 can (15 ounces) chickpeas, drained and rinsed
- 1 can (14.5 ounces) diced tomatoes
- 4 cups vegetable broth
- 1 small sweet potato, peeled and diced
- 1/2 teaspoon sea salt
- 1/4 teaspoon black pepper
- 1 cup chopped spinach or kale
- Juice of 1/2 lemon
- Fresh cilantro

In a large pot, heat the olive oil over medium heat. Add the diced onion and cook until translucent, about 5 minutes. Add the minced garlic and cook for another minute.

Stir in the ground cumin, coriander, turmeric, cayenne pepper, and smoked paprika. Cook for 1-2 minutes until fragrant.

Add the chickpeas and diced tomatoes to the pot. Stir well to coat them with the spices.

Pour in the vegetable broth and add the diced sweet potato. Bring the soup to a boil, then reduce the heat and let it simmer for about 20-25 minutes, or until the sweet potato is tender.

Stir in the chopped spinach or kale, if using, and let it wilt into the soup for about 2-3 minutes.

Season the soup with salt and black pepper to taste. Serve hot, with a squeeze of fresh lemon juice and a sprinkle of cilantro, if desired..

Cauliflower and Leek Soup

Gluten-Free: Yes

Dairy-Free: Yes

Vegan: Yes

Prep Time: 10 minutes Cooking Time: 30 minutes Total Time: 40 minutes Serving Size: 1 cup (about 8 ounces)

Calories: 120

Fat: 5g

Protein: 4g

Carbohydrates: 16g

Fiber: 5g

Sugars: 4g

- 1 medium head of cauliflower, chopped into florets
- 2 large leeks, white and light green parts only, sliced
- 3 cloves garlic, minced
- 4 cups vegetable broth (ensure gluten-free if needed)
- 1 tablespoon olive oil
- 1 teaspoon ground turmeric
- 1/2 teaspoon ground cumin
- 1/4 teaspoon ground black pepper
- Salt
- Fresh parsley or chives

Wash and chop the cauliflower into small florets. Slice the leeks and rinse them thoroughly to remove any grit.

In a large pot, heat the olive oil over medium heat. Add the sliced leeks and garlic, and sauté until the leeks are soft, about 5 minutes.

Add the cauliflower florets to the pot along with the turmeric, cumin, black pepper, and a pinch of salt. Stir to coat the vegetables with the spices.

Pour in the vegetable broth and bring the mixture to a boil. Reduce the heat to low, cover the pot, and let it simmer for about 20 minutes, or until the cauliflower is tender.

Use an immersion blender to blend the soup until smooth and creamy. Alternatively, you can carefully transfer the soup in batches to a blender and blend until smooth.

Taste and adjust the seasoning with more salt if needed.

Ladle the soup into bowls and garnish with fresh parsley or chives if desired.

Pumpkin and Coconut Milk Soup

Gluten-Free: Yes

Dairy-Free: Yes

Vegan: Yes

Prep Time: 10 minutes Cooking Time: 30 minutes Total Time: 40 minutes Serving Size: 1 bowl (about 1 cup)

Calories: 200

Fat: 16g

Protein: 2g

Carbohydrates: 15g

Fiber: 3g

Sugars: 6g

- 1 tablespoon coconut oil
- 1 small onion, diced
- 2 cloves garlic, minced
- 1 teaspoon fresh ginger, grated
- 1 teaspoon ground turmeric
- 1/2 teaspoon ground cumin
- 1/4 teaspoon ground cinnamon
- 4 cups pumpkin puree or 1 small pumpkin, peeled, seeded, and cubed
- 3 cups vegetable broth
- 1 can (14 ounces) full-fat coconut milk
- Salt and pepper to taste
- 1 tablespoon fresh lime juice
- Fresh cilantro

In a large pot, heat the coconut oil over medium heat. Add the diced onion and sauté until soft and translucent, about 5 minutes. Add the garlic, ginger, turmeric, cumin, and cinnamon, and cook for another minute until fragrant.

Stir in the pumpkin puree or cubed pumpkin, and cook for 2-3 minutes, allowing the flavors to blend.

Pour in the vegetable broth, bring to a boil, then reduce the heat and let it simmer for about 20 minutes, or until the pumpkin is tender (if using cubed pumpkin).

Using an immersion blender, blend the soup until smooth. Alternatively, transfer the soup to a blender and blend in batches, then return it to the pot.

Stir in the coconut milk and lime juice, and season with salt and pepper to taste. Simmer for another 5 minutes until the soup is heated through.

Ladle the soup into bowls and garnish with fresh cilantro, if desired. Serve warm.

CHAPTER 11

CONDIMENTS, DRESSING AND SAUCES

Turmeric Mustard

Gluten-Free: Yes

Dairy-Free: Yes

Vegan: Yes

Prep Time: 5 minutes Serving Size: 1 tablespoon (about 20 servings per batch)

(per serving, 1 tablespoon):

Calories: 10

Fat: 0.5g

Protein: 0.5g

Carbohydrates: 1g

Fiber: 0.5g

Sugars: 0.5g

1/2 cup yellow mustard seeds

1/2 cup apple cider vinegar

1/4 cup water

1 tablespoon ground turmeric

1 teaspoon sea salt

1/2 teaspoon ground black pepper

1 tablespoon honey or maple syrup

Place the mustard seeds in a bowl and cover with apple cider vinegar and water. Let them soak for at least 4 hours or overnight. This softens the seeds and makes them easier to blend.

Add the soaked mustard seeds (along with any remaining liquid) to a blender or food processor. Add the turmeric, sea salt, black pepper, and honey/maple syrup (if using).

Blend until the mixture reaches your desired consistency. You can make it smooth or leave it a bit grainy for texture.

If the mustard is too thick, add a bit more water or apple cider vinegar to reach your preferred consistency.

Transfer the mustard to a glass jar and refrigerate. The flavor will develop further after a few days.

Avocado Mayo

Gluten-Free: Yes

Dairy-Free: Yes

Vegan: Yes

Prep Time: 10 minutes Serving Size: 2 tablespoons

1 ripe avocado

1 tablespoon lemon juice or apple cider vinegar

1/2 teaspoon Dijon mustard

1/4 cup olive oil or avocado oil

Salt

Black pepper

(per 2-tablespoon serving):

Calories: 120

Fat: 11g

Protein: 1g

Carbohydrates: 6g

Fiber: 4g

Sugars: 1g

Cut the avocado in half, remove the pit, and scoop the flesh into a food processor or blender.

Add lemon juice, Dijon mustard (if using), and a pinch of salt and pepper to the avocado.

With the food processor or blender running, slowly stream in the olive oil or avocado oil until the mixture is smooth and creamy.

Taste and adjust seasoning with additional salt, pepper, or lemon juice if needed.

Transfer the avocado mayo to a container with a tight-fitting lid. Store in the refrigerator for up to 1 week.

Beet Ketchup

Gluten-Free: Yes

Dairy-Free: Yes

Vegan: Yes

Prep Time: 10 minutes Cooking Time: 30 minutes Total Time: 40 minutes Serving Size: 2 tablespoons (about 1/8 cup)

(per 2 tablespoons):

Calories: 30

Fat: 1g

Protein: 0.5g

Carbohydrates: 7g

Fiber: 1g

Sugars: 5g

- 2 medium beets, peeled and chopped
- 1/2 cup tomato paste
- 1/4 cup apple cider vinegar
- 1/4 cup water
- 2 tablespoons maple syrup or honey
- 1 tablespoon olive oil
- 1 teaspoon ground turmeric
- 1/2 teaspoon ground cinnamon
- 1/4 teaspoon ground ginger
- 1/4 teaspoon garlic powder
- 1/4 teaspoon onion powder
- 1/4 teaspoon salt
- A pinch of black pepper

In a medium saucepan, cover the chopped beets with water. Bring to a boil over high heat, then reduce heat to medium and simmer until beets are tender, about 15-20 minutes. Drain and let cool slightly.

In a blender or food processor, blend the cooked beets until smooth. Set aside.

In the same saucepan, heat the olive oil over medium heat. Add the tomato paste, apple cider vinegar, and water. Stir until well combined.

Stir in the maple syrup or honey, turmeric, cinnamon, ginger, garlic powder, onion powder, salt, and black pepper. Mix well.

Add the blended beets to the saucepan. Stir and let the mixture simmer over low heat for about 10-15 minutes, stirring occasionally

until the ketchup thickens to your desired consistency.

Let the beet ketchup cool before transferring it to an airtight container. Store in the refrigerator for up to 2 weeks.

Spicy Mango Chutney

Gluten-Free: Yes

Dairy-Free: Yes

Vegan: Yes

Prep Time: 10 minutes Cooking Time: 20 minutes Total Time: 30 minutes Serving Size: 2 tablespoons (about 30 grams)

(per serving, 2 tablespoons):

Calories: 40

Fat: 1.5g

Protein: 0.5g

Carbohydrates: 7g

Fiber: 1g

Sugars: 6g

- 2 ripe mangoes, peeled and diced
- 1 small onion, finely chopped
- 1 red chili, finely chopped
- 1/4 cup apple cider vinegar
- 1/4 cup brown sugar or coconut sugar
- 1 tablespoon fresh ginger, minced
- 1/2 teaspoon ground cumin
- 1/2 teaspoon ground coriander
- 1/4 teaspoon ground turmeric
- 1/4 teaspoon ground cinnamon
- 1/4 teaspoon salt
- 1 tablespoon olive oil

Peel and dice the mangoes, finely chop the onion and chili, and mince the ginger.

In a medium saucepan, heat the olive oil over medium heat. Add the onion and chili, cooking until the onion becomes translucent.

Stir in the ginger, cumin, coriander, turmeric, cinnamon, and salt. Cook for about 1 minute, allowing the spices to become fragrant.

Add the diced mangoes, apple cider vinegar, and brown sugar to the saucepan. Stir to combine.

Bring the mixture to a boil, then reduce the heat and let it simmer for 15-20 minutes, or until the mangoes are soft and the chutney has thickened.

Remove from heat and let the chutney cool. Transfer to a clean jar and store in the refrigerator for up to 2 weeks.

Lemon-Tahini Dressing

Gluten-Free: Yes

Dairy-Free: Yes

Vegan: Yes

Prep Time: 5 minutes Serving Size: 2 tablespoons (about 30 ml)

(per 2 tablespoons):

Calories: 90

Fat: 8g

Protein: 2g

Carbohydrates: 4g

Fiber: 1g

Sugars: 0g

1/4 cup tahini (sesame seed paste)

2 tablespoons fresh lemon juice

1 tablespoon extra virgin olive oil

1 clove garlic, minced

1 tablespoon water

1/2 teaspoon ground cumin

Salt and black pepper

In a small bowl, whisk together the tahini, lemon juice, olive oil, minced garlic, and ground cumin (if using).

Add water a little at a time, whisking until the dressing reaches your desired consistency. If it's too thick, add more water; if it's too thin, add more tahini.

Season with salt and black pepper to taste. Adjust the lemon juice or garlic if needed.

Use immediately or store in an airtight container in the refrigerator for up to one week.

Ginger-Miso Dressing

Gluten-Free: No

Dairy-Free: Yes

Vegan: Yes

Prep Time: 10 minutes **Serving Size:** 2 tablespoons

- 2 tablespoons white miso paste
- 1 tablespoon grated fresh ginger
- 2 tablespoons rice vinegar
- 1 tablespoon tamari (gluten-free soy sauce) or regular soy sauce
- 1 tablespoon sesame oil
- 1 teaspoon maple syrup or honey
- 1 clove garlic, minced
- 1 tablespoon water

(per serving, 2 tablespoons):

Calories: 40

Fat: 2g

Protein: 1g

Carbohydrates: 4g

Fiber: 0g

Sugars: 2g

In a small bowl, whisk together the miso paste, grated ginger, rice vinegar, tamari (or soy sauce), sesame oil, and maple syrup or honey (if using).

Stir in the minced garlic.

Add water a little at a time, whisking until you reach your desired consistency.

Use as a salad dressing or store in an airtight container in the refrigerator for up to a week.

Turmeric Tahini Sauce

Gluten-Free: Yes

Dairy-Free: Yes

Vegan: Yes

Prep Time: 5 minutes Serving Size: 2 tablespoons

- 1/2 cup tahini (sesame seed paste)
- 1 tablespoon freshly squeezed lemon juice
- 1 teaspoon ground turmeric
- 1/2 teaspoon ground cumin
- 1/4 teaspoon garlic powder
- 1/4 teaspoon ground ginger
- 1/4 teaspoon black pepper
- 2-3 tablespoons water
- Salt

(per serving, 2 tablespoons):

- Calories: 90
- Fat: 8g
- Protein: 3g
- Carbohydrates: 4g
- Fiber: 2g
- Sugars: 1g

In a small bowl, mix together the tahini, lemon juice, turmeric, cumin, garlic powder, ginger, and black pepper.

Gradually add water, one tablespoon at a time, until you reach your desired consistency. The sauce should be smooth and pourable.

Taste and adjust salt if needed.

Use or store in an airtight container in the refrigerator for up to one week.

Cilantro-Lime Sauce

Gluten-Free: Yes

Dairy-Free: Yes

Vegan: Yes

Prep Time: 10 minutes Serving Size: 2 tablespoons (about 30 grams)

1 cup fresh cilantro leaves, packed

1/4 cup lime juice (about 2 limes)

(per 2 tablespoons):

1/4 cup olive oil

Calories: 80

2 garlic cloves

Fat: 9g

1/2 teaspoon ground cumin

Protein: 0g

1/4 teaspoon salt

Carbohydrates: 1g

1/4 teaspoon black pepper

Fiber: 0g

Sugars: 0g

Wash the cilantro leaves thoroughly and peel the garlic cloves.

In a blender or food processor, combine the cilantro, lime juice, olive oil, garlic, cumin, salt, and black pepper.

Blend until the mixture is smooth and well combined. Scrape down the sides as needed.

Taste and adjust seasoning if needed, adding more salt or lime juice according to preference.

Transfer the sauce to a container. It can be used immediately or stored in the refrigerator for up to 1 week.

Ginger-Sesame Sauce

Gluten-Free: Yes

Dairy-Free: Yes

Vegan: Yes

Prep Time: 10 minutes Serving Size: 2 tablespoons

(per 2 tablespoons):

Calories: 80

Fat: 8g

Protein: 1g

Carbohydrates: 3g

Fiber: 0g

Sugars: 2g

1/4 cup sesame oil

2 tablespoons gluten-free tamari or soy sauce (use tamari for gluten-free)

1 tablespoon rice vinegar

1 tablespoon honey or maple syrup

1 tablespoon freshly grated ginger

1 garlic clove, minced

1 teaspoon sesame seeds

1/4 teaspoon ground black pepper

In a small bowl, whisk together the sesame oil, tamari (or soy sauce), rice vinegar, and honey (or maple syrup).

Stir in the freshly grated ginger, minced garlic, and black pepper.

Sprinkle sesame seeds on top if desired.

Use immediately or store in an airtight container in the refrigerator for up to 1 week.

Cashew Cream Sauce

Gluten-Free: Yes

Dairy-Free: Yes **Prep Time:** 10 minutes **Serving Size:** 1/4 cup

Vegan: Yes

1 cup raw cashews, soaked for at least 2 hours or overnight

1/2 cup water

1 tablespoon lemon juice

1 tablespoon nutritional yeast

1 garlic clove

1/2 teaspoon salt (or to taste)

1/4 teaspoon ground turmeric

(per 1/4 cup serving):

Calories: 90

Fat: 7g

Protein: 3g

Carbohydrates: 7g

Fiber: 1g

Sugars: 1g

Drain and rinse the soaked cashews.

In a high-speed blender, combine the soaked cashews, water, lemon juice, nutritional yeast, garlic clove, salt, and turmeric (if using).

Blend on high until the mixture is completely smooth and creamy. You can add more water if you prefer a thinner sauce.

Taste and adjust the seasoning as needed.

Use immediately or store in an airtight container in the refrigerator for up to 5 days.

12: Better Sleep, Minimized Stress Levels and Physical Activity

Better Sleep: The Foundation of Health

I used to be a night owl, frequently staying up late reading through social media or binge-watching TV series. I didn't know how much this was harming my entire health until I made a deliberate effort to prioritize sleep.

Now, I try for 7-8 hours of great sleep each night. I've created a constant sleep regimen, going to bed and getting up at the same time every day, including on weekends. This has helped adjust my body's internal schedule, making it simpler to go asleep and wake up naturally.

I've also devised a peaceful nighttime regimen. About an hour before bed, I reduce the lights and avoid screens. Instead, I read a book, perform moderate yoga, or do some light stretching. I've discovered that this helps convey to my body that it's time to wind down.

The effect on my inflammation levels has been evident. I wake up feeling invigorated instead of drowsy, and the continual low-grade pains I used to encounter have greatly lessened. My energy levels throughout the day have increased, and I'm more suited to manage stress.

Minimizing Stress: A Daily Practice

Learning to manage and limit stress has been a game-changer for me.

I've included various stress-reduction tactics into my regular practice. Meditation has proven extremely beneficial. I start each morning with a 10-minute meditation practice, which helps create a peaceful tone for the day. When I sense tension increasing throughout the day, I take a few minutes for deep breathing exercises.

I've also learned to say "no" more frequently, creating limits to safeguard my time and energy. This has helped decrease the continual sensation of being overwhelmed that used to torment me.

Another important shift has been reducing my exposure to unpleasant news and social media. While I keep informed, I no longer allow myself to become trapped in the loop of frequent news intake that was raising my stress levels.

The impact on my inflammation levels has been remarkable. The continual strain I used to carry in my shoulders and jaw has alleviated. I've seen less stress-related breakouts, and my digestion has improved dramatically.

Physical Activity: Moving Towards Health

Before my lifestyle modifications, my concept of exercise was walking from my vehicle to my workplace. Now, regular physical exercise is a non-negotiable component of my day.

I start most mornings with a quick 30-minute stroll. This not only gets my blood flowing but also exposes me to morning sunshine, which helps reset my circadian cycle. On days when I can't go outdoors, I utilize a treadmill or do some yoga inside.

Three times a week, I undertake strength training exercises. I began modestly, with bodyweight workouts and light weights, gradually increasing the intensity as I became stronger. This has helped develop muscle, which I've discovered has a part in lowering general inflammation in the body.

I've also found the thrill of dancing. Twice a week, I take a dancing class. It's a great method to get cardiac exercise, plus the social component contributes to my general well-being.

The effect on my inflammation levels has been tremendous. The persistent joint discomfort I used to feel has all but vanished. My energy levels have risen, and I feel I'm a lot more resilient to disease.

Bringing It All Together

What I've learned on this path is that sleep, stress management, and physical exercise are all interrelated. When I sleep better, I'm more able to manage stress and more eager to exercise. When I exercise consistently, I sleep better and feel less stressed. And when I handle my stress efficiently, I sleep better and have more energy for physical exercise.

Living an inflammation-free life isn't about perfection. There are still days when I don't get enough sleep, moments when stress gets the better of me, or weeks when I'm not as active as I'd want to be. But by continuously addressing these three areas, I've established a lifestyle that supports my body in reducing inflammation.

The improvements in how I feel have been remarkable. The daily exhaustion, pains, and mental fog that I used to consider usual are now uncommon occurrences. I feel more bright, clear-headed, and resilient than I have in years.

If you're battling with inflammation, I recommend you look at your sleep patterns, stress levels, and physical activity. Small, persistent adjustments in these areas may lead to big gains in your overall health and well-being.

Food Elimination and Reintroduction

This is a systematic strategy used to detect possible dietary sensitivities or intolerances that may be related to inflammation in the body. This technique entails temporarily omitting particular items from your diet and then progressively returning them while monitoring your body's responses.

The theory behind food removal and reintroduction is that some foods may cause inflammatory reactions in certain people. These reactions may be subtle and cumulative, making them difficult to recognize without an organized method. By eliminating possible trigger foods and then returning them one at a time, you may more readily pinpoint which foods may be creating troubles for you specifically.

Common Inflammatory Trigger Foods

While individual responses can vary, some common foods that are often eliminated in this process include:

1. Dairy products
2. Gluten-containing grains
3. Soy
4. Eggs
5. Nuts and seeds
6. Nightshade vegetables (tomatoes, peppers, eggplants, potatoes)
7. Citrus fruits
8. Corn
9. Sugar and artificial sweeteners
10. Processed foods and additives

The Elimination Phase

Step 1: Preparation

Before beginning the elimination phase:

- Consult with a healthcare provider or registered dietitian to ensure this approach is appropriate for you.
- Plan your meals for the elimination period to ensure you're still getting all necessary nutrients
- Clean out your pantry and fridge of foods you'll be eliminating.
- Stock up on allowed foods.
- Keep a food and symptom journal throughout the process.

Step 2: Elimination

- Remove all potential trigger foods from your diet for a set period, typically 2-4 weeks.

- During this time, focus on consuming a variety of anti-inflammatory foods such as
    i. Leafy green vegetable
    ii. Berries and other low-sugar fruits
    iii. Fatty fish rich in omega-3s
    iv. Lean proteins
    v. Healthy fats like olive oil and avocado
    vi. Herbs and spices known for their anti-inflammatory properties

Step 3: Observation

- Pay close attention to how you feel during the elimination phase.
- Note any changes in symptoms such as digestive issues, skin conditions, energy levels, mood, or any chronic health conditions you may have
- It's common to experience some withdrawal symptoms in the first few days, especially if you've eliminated sugar or caffeine.

The Reintroduction Phase

Step 1: Planning

- Create a reintroduction schedule, typically reintroducing one food group every 3-7 days.
- Start with foods you suspect are least likely to cause a reaction.

Step 2: Reintroduction

- Reintroduce one food at a time in its purest form. For example, if reintroducing dairy, start with plain, organic milk rather than cheese or yogurt.
- Consume a small amount of the food on day one, a larger amount on day two, and observe for the next 2-5 days without consuming the food again.

Step 3: Monitoring

- Carefully observe and record any symptoms that occur after reintroducing a food.
- Symptoms to watch for include:
    i. Digestive issues (bloating, gas, diarrhea, constipation)

    ii. Skin reactions (rashes, acne, eczema flare-ups)
    iii. Headaches or migraines
    iv. Joint pain or muscle aches
    v. Fatigue or changes in energy levels
    vi. Mood changes
    vii. Sinus congestion or runny nose
    viii. Changes in sleep patterns

Step 4: Decision Making

- If you experience no negative reactions, you can likely include this food in your diet
- If you experience a reaction, consider eliminating this food from your diet long-term or discuss further steps with your healthcare provider.

Step 5: Continue the Process

- Move on to the next food group, following the same process.
- Continue until you've tested all the eliminated foods.

Your Anti-Inflammatory Diet: How to Apply the Findings

After you've finished the procedure of removing and then reintroducing:

1. Use your data to create a customized eating plan that reduces inflammation.
2. Make it a point to include a diverse range of foods that are anti-inflammatory and that you can eat without any problems.
3. Consider rotating foods to avoid acquiring new sensitivities.
4. Continue to pay attention to how various meals make you feel

Long-Term Management

Now that you know what foods set off your allergy

- First, remember that tolerances are fluid and should be reevaluated from time to time.
- Pay attention to your digestive system by eating prebiotic and probiotic foods; this could help you build a tolerance to certain meals.
- You should think about collaborating with a healthcare professional to deal with the underlying reasons of your body's inflammation.
- Keep in mind that inflammation management is not the only thing that relies on sleep, physical exercise, and stress. Along with your nutrition, you should also focus on these other parts of your lifestyle.

30 DAYS MEAL PLAN

Week 1

Day 1

- Breakfast: Avocado-Banana Smoothie
- Lunch: Kale and Quinoa Salad
- Dinner: Ginger-Turmeric Beef Stir-Fry
- Snack: Golden Milk Energy Balls

Day 2

- Breakfast: Lemon-Blueberry Ricotta Pancakes
- Lunch: Chicken and Spinach Wrap
- Dinner: Lemon-Dill Baked Trout
- Snack: Nut Butter Apple Slices

Day 3

- Breakfast: Blueberry-Spinach Smoothie
- Lunch: Sweet Potato and Black Bean Salad
- Dinner: Herb-Roasted Pork Tenderloin with Garlic Green Beans
- Snack: Beetroot Smoothie

Day 4

- Breakfast: Chia Seed Pancakes
- Lunch: Caprese-Stuffed Portobello Mushrooms
- Dinner: Miso-Glazed Salmon with Cabbage and Kale Soup
- Snack: Cucumber and Hummus Bites

Day 5

- Breakfast: Avocado & Kale Omelet
- Lunch: Mediterranean Lentil Salad
- Dinner: Turmeric-Spiced Shrimp with Cauliflower Rice Salad
- Snack: Spinach and Berry Salad

Day 6

- Breakfast: Spinach & Egg Scramble
- Lunch: Sweet Potato-Black Bean Tacos
- Dinner: Chicken and Sweet Potato Stew
- Snack: Turmeric Roasted Chickpeas

Day 7

- Breakfast: Smoked Salmon & Omelet
- Lunch: Vegan Buddha Bowl
- Dinner: Mushroom Barley Soup
- Snack: Garlic-Lemon Scallops

Week 2

Day 8

- Breakfast: Green Smoothie
- Lunch: Herring with Beet Salad
- Dinner: Lemon-Herb Roasted Chicken with Sweet Potato Fries
- Snack: Avocado Hummus with Carrot and Celery Sticks

Day 9

- Breakfast: Pumpkin Spice Pancakes
- Lunch: Tofu and Veggie Wrap
- Dinner: Rosemary Garlic Lamb Chops with Spinach and Berry Salad
- Snack: Berry-Kefir Smoothie

Day 10

- Breakfast: Mushroom & Spinach Frittata
- Lunch: Spiced Turkey Meatballs with Cilantro-Lime Sauce
- Dinner: Mackerel and Olive Relish with Arugula and Beet Salad
- Snack: Sweet Potato Chips

Day 11

- Breakfast: Banana Oat Pancakes
- Lunch: Chickpea and Spinach Curry
- Dinner: Quinoa Vegetable Soup
- Snack: Turmeric Popcorn

Day 12

- Breakfast: Cherry-Mocha Smoothie
- Lunch: Seaweed and Tuna Wrap
- Dinner: Mushroom Risotto with Turmeric Tahini Sauce
- Snack: Blueberry Almond Bites

Day 13

- Breakfast: Southwestern Waffle with Eggs
- Lunch: Sardine Salad
- Dinner: Spicy Chicken Lettuce Wraps
- Snack: Avocado Mayo with Carrot and Celery Sticks

Day 14

- Breakfast: Golden Milk
- Lunch: Vegan Lentil Soup
- Dinner: Vegetable Paella with Ginger-Miso Dressing
- Snack: Pineapple-Ginger Smoothie

Week 3

Day 15

- Breakfast: Avocado & Kale Omelet
- Lunch: Sweet Potato and Black Bean Salad
- Dinner: Turmeric Chicken Soup
- Snack: Cashew Cream Sauce with Cucumber and Hummus Bites

Day 16

- Breakfast: Beetroot Smoothie
- Lunch: Caprese-Stuffed Portobello Mushrooms
- Dinner: Garlic-Lemon Scallops with Garlic Green Beans
- Snack: Chia Seed Pancakes

Day 17

- Breakfast: Green Smoothie
- Lunch: Chicken and Spinach Wrap
- Dinner: Miso Soup with Tofu and Mushroom Barley Soup
- Snack: Nut Butter Apple Slices

Day 18

- Breakfast: Pumpkin Spice Pancakes
- Lunch: Chickpea and Spinach Curry
- Dinner: Lentil and Spinach Stew
- Snack: Turmeric Mustard with Carrot and Celery Sticks

Day 19

- Breakfast: Smoked Salmon & Omelet
- Lunch: Arugula and Beet Salad
- Dinner: Beef and Vegetable Kebabs with Cilantro-Lime Sauce
- Snack: Spinach and Berry Salad

Day 20

- Breakfast: Golden Milk
- Lunch: Vegan Buddha Bowl
- Dinner: Ginger-Garlic Chicken Stir-Fry with Cauliflower Rice Salad
- Snack: Blueberry Almond Bites

Day 21

- Breakfast: Turmeric Latte
- Lunch: Sweet Potato-Black Bean Tacos
- Dinner: Pumpkin and Coconut Milk Soup with Rosemary Garlic Lamb Chops
- Snack: Pineapple-Ginger Smoothie

Week 4

Day 22

- Breakfast: Cherry-Mocha Smoothie
- Lunch: Tofu and Veggie Wrap
- Dinner: Lemon-Dill Baked Trout with Arugula and Beet Salad
- Snack: Garlic Green Beans

Day 23

- Breakfast: Banana Oat Pancakes
- Lunch: Mediterranean Lentil Salad
- Dinner: Herb-Roasted Pork Tenderloin with Ginger-Turmeric Beef Stir-Fry
- Snack: Avocado Hummus with Carrot and Celery Sticks

Day 24

- Breakfast: Avocado-Banana Smoothie
- Lunch: Spinach and Berry Salad
- Dinner: Spicy Chickpea Soup with Sweet Potato Fries
- Snack: Golden Milk Energy Balls

Day 25

- Breakfast: Mushroom & Spinach Frittata
- Lunch: Spiced Turkey Meatballs with Turmeric Tahini Sauce
- Dinner: Miso-Glazed Salmon with Quinoa Vegetable Soup
- Snack: Sweet Potato Chips

Day 26

- Breakfast: Green Smoothie
- Lunch: Sardine Salad
- Dinner: Vegetable Paella with Ginger-Miso Dressing
- Snack: Cashew Cream Sauce with Cucumber and Hummus Bites

Day 27

- Breakfast: Lemon-Blueberry Ricotta Pancakes
- Lunch: Chicken and Spinach Wrap
- Dinner: Turmeric-Spiced Shrimp with Cauliflower Rice Salad
- Snack: Blueberry Almond Bites

Day 28

- Breakfast: Turmeric Latte
- Lunch: Herring with Beet Salad
- Dinner: Lemon-Herb Roasted Chicken with Sweet Potato Fries
- Snack: Pineapple-Ginger Smoothie

Day 29

- Breakfast: Avocado & Kale Omelet
- Lunch: Vegan Lentil Soup
- Dinner: Mushroom Risotto with Cilantro-Lime Sauce
- Snack: Turmeric Roasted Chickpeas

Day 30

- Breakfast: Beetroot Smoothie
- Lunch: Sweet Potato and Black Bean Salad
- Dinner: Lemon-Dill Baked Trout with Garlic Green Beans
- Snack: Nut Butter Apple Slices

RECIPE INDEX

A

Avocado Mayo168

Arugula and Beet Salad93

Avocado Hummus76

Avocado & Kale Omelet56

Avocado-Banana Smoothie49

B

Beet Ketchup169

Beef and Vegetable Kebabs146

Blackened Catfish126

Blueberry Almond Bites87

Beetroot Smoothie50

Berry-Kefir Smoothie44

Blueberry-Spinach Smoothie52

Banana Oat Pancakes 67

C

Cabbage and Kale Soup 154

Chicken and Sweet Potato Stew 138

Caprese-Stuffed Portobello Mushrooms 104

Cauliflower Rice Salad 95

Cucumber and Hummus Bites 78

Chia Seed Pancakes 72

Cherry-Mocha Smoothie 47

Carrot and Celery Sticks with Guacamole 81

Chicken and Spinach Wrap 98

Chickpea and Spinach Curry 112

Cauliflower and Leek Soup 162

Cilantro-Lime Sauce 176

Cashew Cream Sauce 178

E

Egg & Veggie Burrito 63

Egg Salad Avocado Toast 58

G

Ginger-Sesame Sauce 177

Ginger-Turmeric Beef Stir-Fry 141

Ginger-Garlic Chicken Stir-Fry 133

Garlic-Lemon Scallops 123

Garlic Green Beans 100

Green Smoothie 51

Golden Milk 48

Golden Milk Energy Balls 79

Ginger-Miso Dressing 174

H

Herb-Roasted Pork Tenderloin 143

Herring with Beet Salad 125

K

Kale and Quinoa Salad 89

L

Lemon-Tahini Dressing 173

Lemon-Herb Roasted Chicken 135

Lemon-Dill Baked Trout 128

Lentil and Spinach Stew 107

Lemon-Blueberry Ricotta Pancakes 71

M

Miso Soup with Tofu 151

Miso-Glazed Salmon 129

Mackerel and Olive Relish 119

Mushroom Risotto 111

Mediterranean Lentil Salad 94

Mushroom & Spinach Frittata 65

Mango-Kale Smoothie 46

Mushroom Barley Soup 158

N

Nut Butter Apple Slices 77

P

Pumpkin and Coconut Milk Soup 164

Pumpkin Spice Pancakes 69

Pineapple-Ginger Smoothie 51

Q

Quinoa Vegetable Soup 152

R

Rosemary Garlic Lamb Chops 140

S

Spinach and Berry Salad 91

Sweet Potato Chips 85

Spinach & Egg Scramble 53

Smoked Salmon & Omelet 60

Southwestern Waffle with Eggs 61

Sweet Potato Waffles 68

Sweet Potato and Black Bean Salad 96

Sweet Potato Fries 102

Sweet Potato-Black Bean Tacos 105

Sardine Salad 121

Spicy Chicken Lettuce Wraps 136

Spiced Turkey Meatballs 145

Seaweed and Tuna Wrap 127

Spicy Mango Chutney 170

Spicy Chickpea Soup 160

T

Turmeric Mustard 167

Turmeric Tahini Sauce 175

Turmeric-Spiced Shrimp 118

Tuna and White Bean Salad 122

Turmeric Chickpea Salad 82

Turmeric Roasted Chickpeas 75

Turmeric Popcorn 87

Turmeric Latte 45

Tofu and Veggie Wrap 99

Turmeric Chicken 131

Turmeric Chicken Soup 149

Turkish Red Lentil Soup 156

V

Vegetable Paella 109

Vegan Buddha Bowl 114

Vegan Lentil Soup 116

References

Cano-Ortiz, A., Laborda-Illanes, A., Plaza-Andrades, I., Del Pozo, A. M., Cuadrado, A. V., De Mora, M. R. C., Leiva-Gea, I., Sanchez-Alcoholado, L., & Queipo-Ortuño, M. I. (2020). Connection between the Gut Microbiome, Systemic Inflammation, Gut Permeability and FOXP3 Expression in Patients with Primary Sjögren's Syndrome. International Journal of Molecular Sciences, 21(22), 8733. https://doi.org/10.3390/ijms21228733

Cherkin, D. C., Sherman, K. J., Balderson, B. H., Cook, A. J., Anderson, M. L., Hawkes, R. J., Hansen, K. E., & Turner, J. A. (2016). Effect of Mindfulness-Based Stress Reduction vs Cognitive Behavioral Therapy or Usual Care on Back Pain and Functional Limitations in Adults With Chronic Low Back Pain. JAMA, 315(12), 1240. https://doi.org/10.1001/jama.2016.2323

D'Aiuto, F., Nibali, L., Parkar, M., Patel, K., Suvan, J., & Donos, N. (2010). Oxidative stress, systemic inflammation, and severe periodontitis. Journal of Dental Research, 89(11), 1241–1246. https://doi.org/10.1177/0022034510375830

Holmes, C., Cunningham, C., Zotova, E., Woolford, J., Dean, C., Kerr, S., Culliford, D., & Perry, V. H. (2009). Systemic inflammation and disease progression in Alzheimer disease. Neurology, 73(10), 768–774. https://doi.org/10.1212/wnl.0b013e3181b6bb95

Kalliomäki, M., Salminen, S., Arvilommi, H., Kero, P., Koskinen, P., & Isolauri, E. (2001). Probiotics in primary prevention of atopic disease: a randomized placebo-controlled trial. The Lancet, 357(9262), 1076–1079. https://doi.org/10.1016/s0140-6736(00)04259-8

Kiecolt-Glaser, J. K., Glaser, R., Shuttleworth, E. C., Dyer, C. S., Ogrocki, P., & Speicher, C. E. (1987). Chronic stress and immunity in family caregivers of Alzheimer's disease victims. Psychosomatic Medicine, 49(5), 523–535. https://doi.org/10.1097/00006842-198709000-00008

O'Leary, K. (2021). Health benefits of fermented foods. Nature Medicine. https://doi.org/10.1038/d41591-021-00053-1

Shah, A. M., Tarfeen, N., Mohamed, H., & Song, Y. (2023). Fermented Foods: Their Health-Promoting Components and Potential Effects on gut microbiota. Fermentation, 9(2), 118. https://doi.org/10.3390/fermentation9020118

Vadell, A. K., Bärebring, L., Hulander, E., Gjertsson, I., Lindqvist, H. M., & Winkvist, A. (2020). Anti-inflammatory Diet In Rheumatoid Arthritis (ADIRA)—a randomized, controlled crossover trial indicating effects on disease activity. American Journal of Clinical Nutrition, 111(6), 1203–1213. https://doi.org/10.1093/ajcn/nqaa019

Woelber, J. P., Gärtner, M., Breuninger, L., Anderson, A., König, D., Hellwig, E., Al-Ahmad, A., Vach, K., Dötsch, A., Ratka-Krüger, P., & Tennert, C. (2019). The influence of an anti-inflammatory diet on gingivitis. A randomized controlled trial. Journal of Clinical Periodontology, 46(4), 481–490. https://doi.org/10.1111/jcpe.13094

Yang, J., Zhang, L., Yu, C., Yang, X., & Wang, H. (2014). Monocyte and macrophage differentiation: circulation inflammatory monocyte as biomarker for inflammatory diseases. Biomarker Research, 2(1). https://doi.org/10.1186/2050-7771-2-1

FOODS ELIMINATION PLAN

TEMPLATE

DATE: 1/9/24 – 30/9/24	
FOODS ELIMINATED	**OBSERVATIONS**

DATE: 1/10/24 – 4/10/24	
FOODS REINTRODUCED	**OBSERVATIONS**

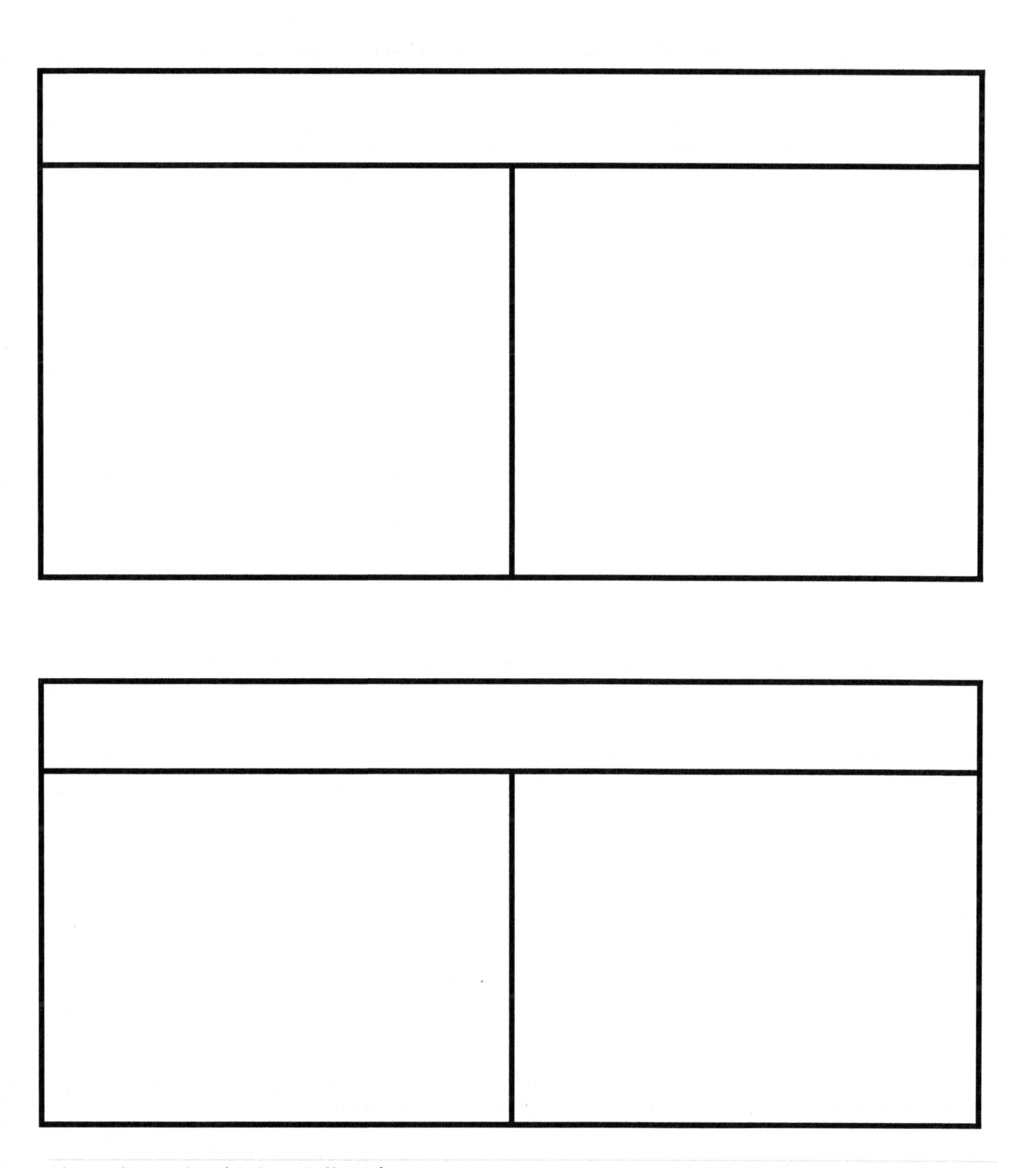

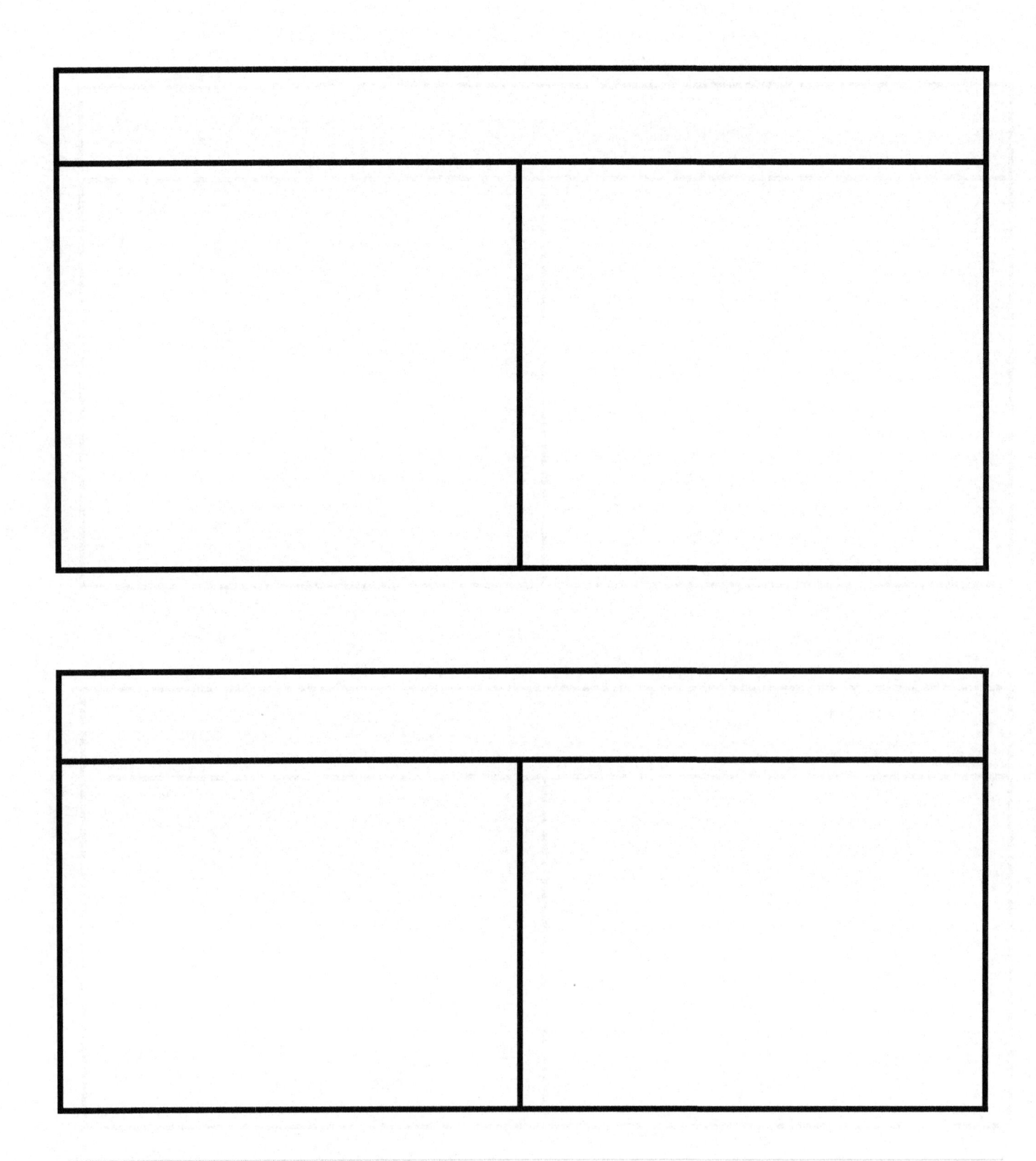

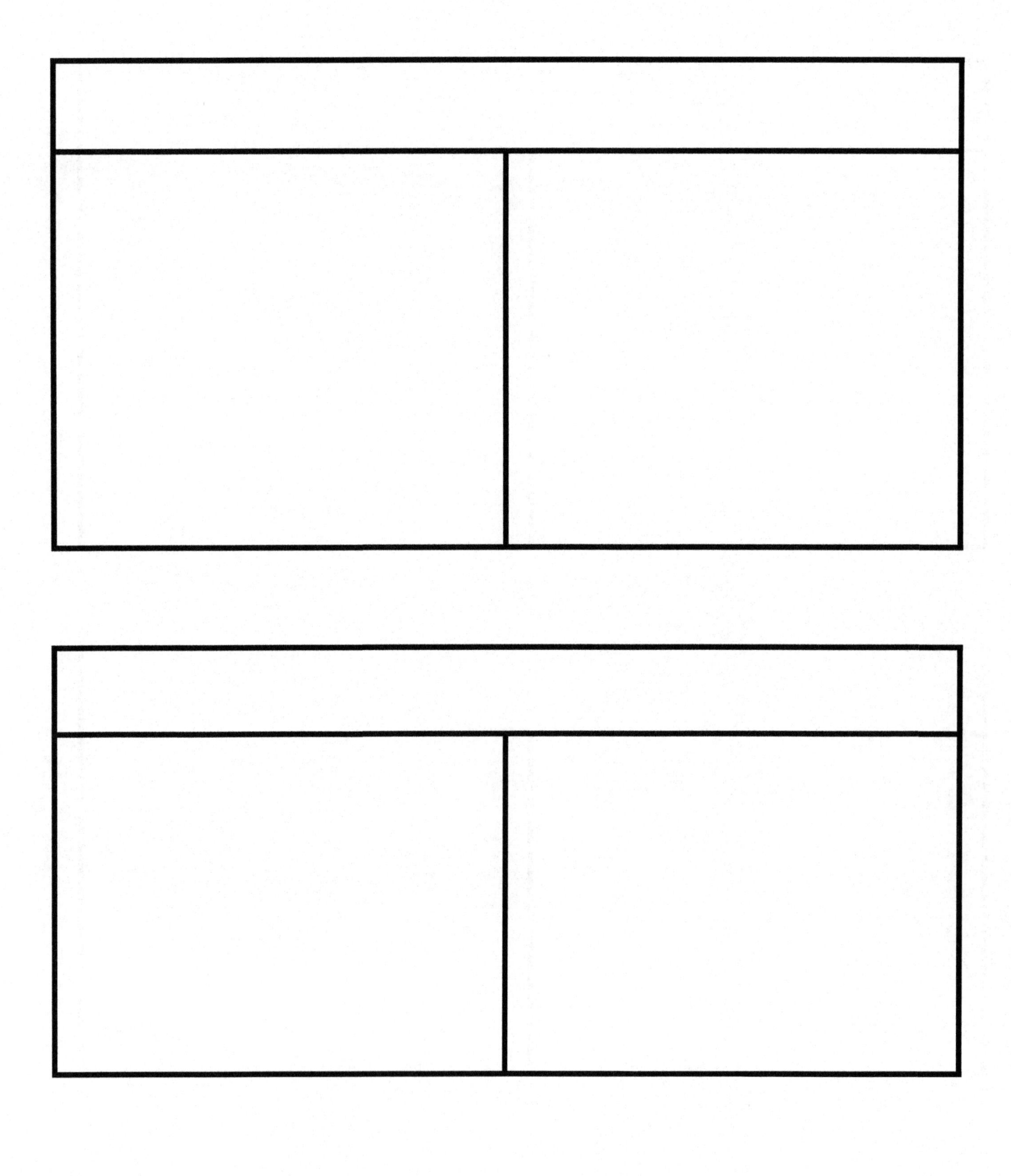

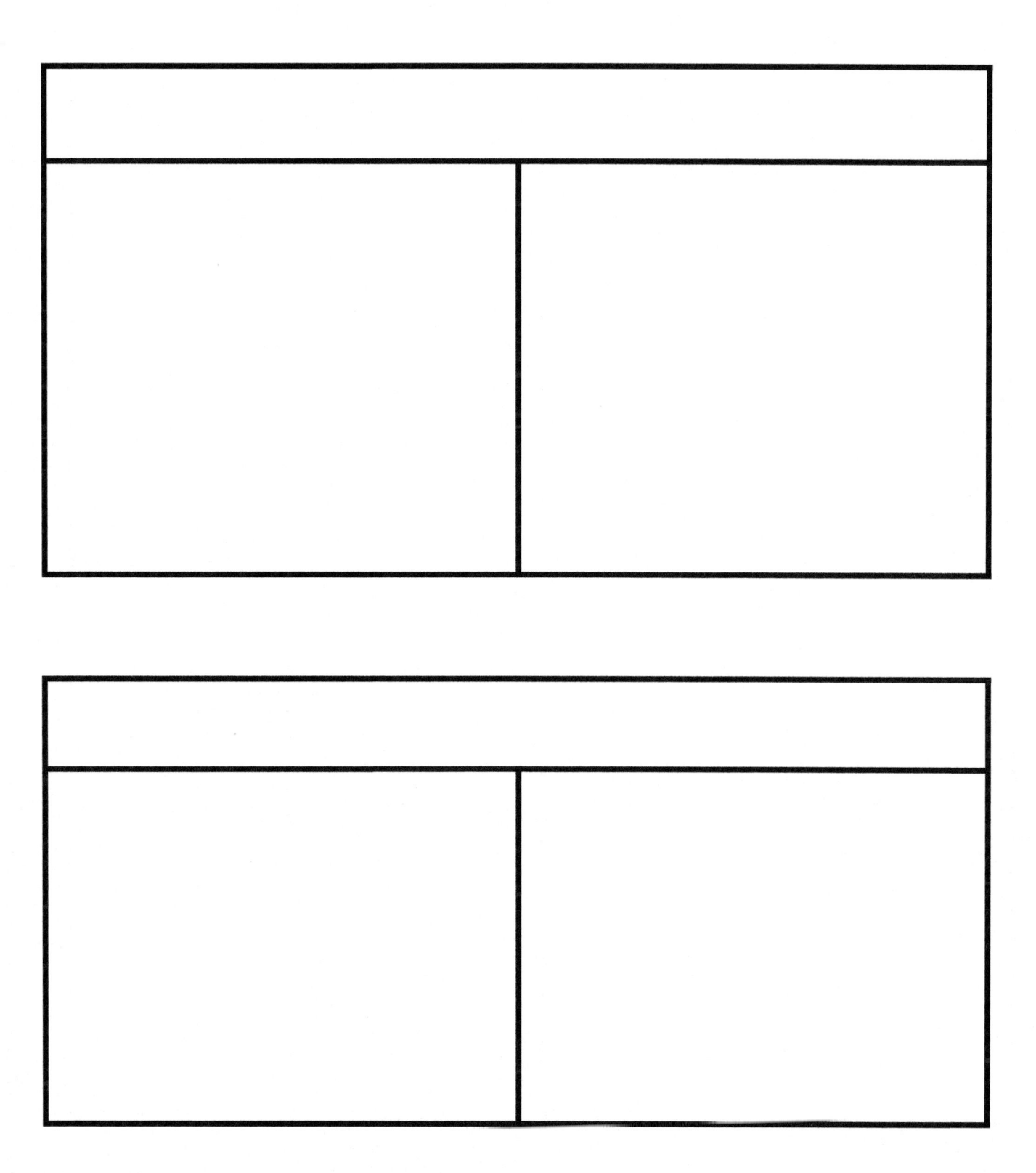

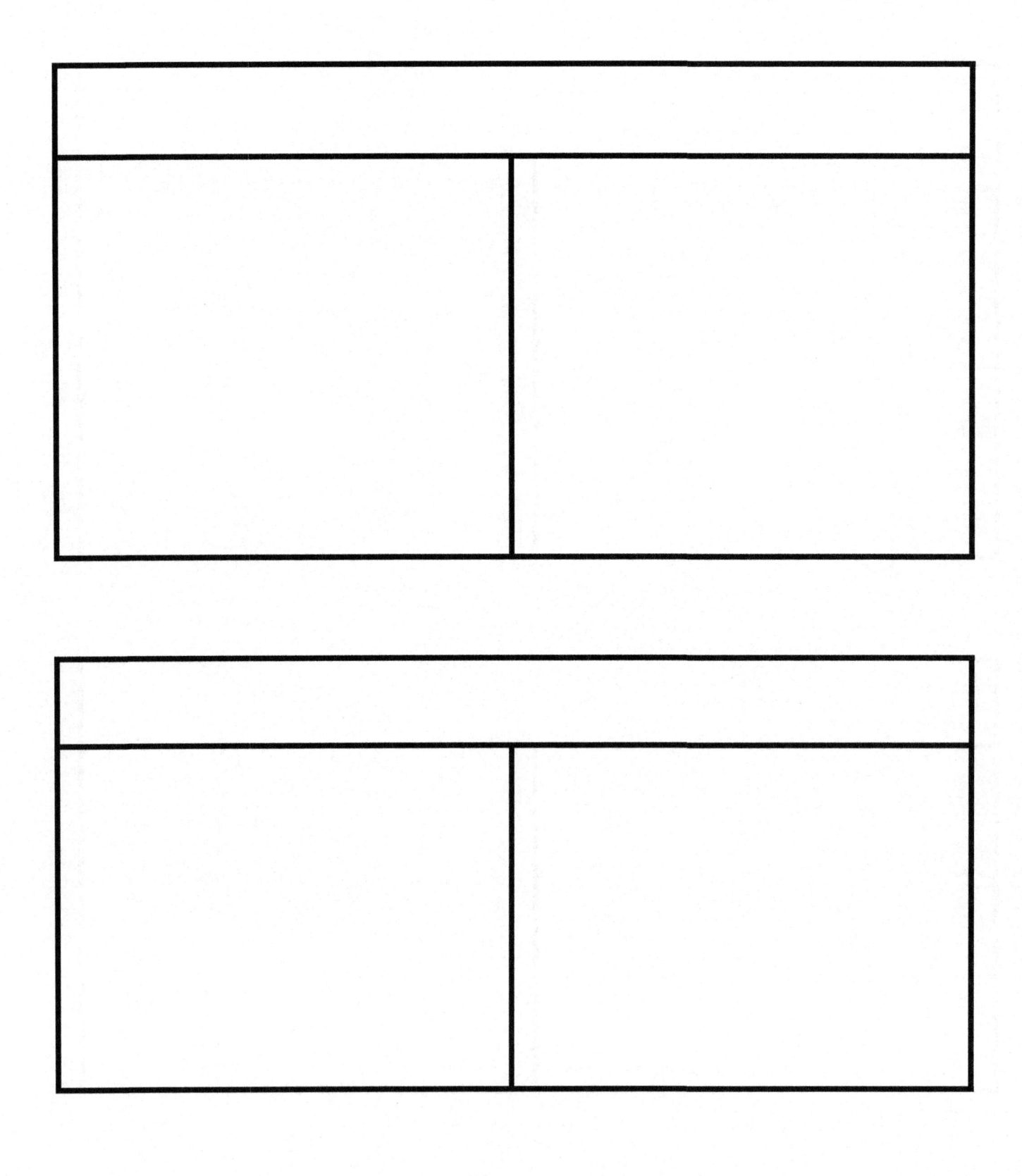

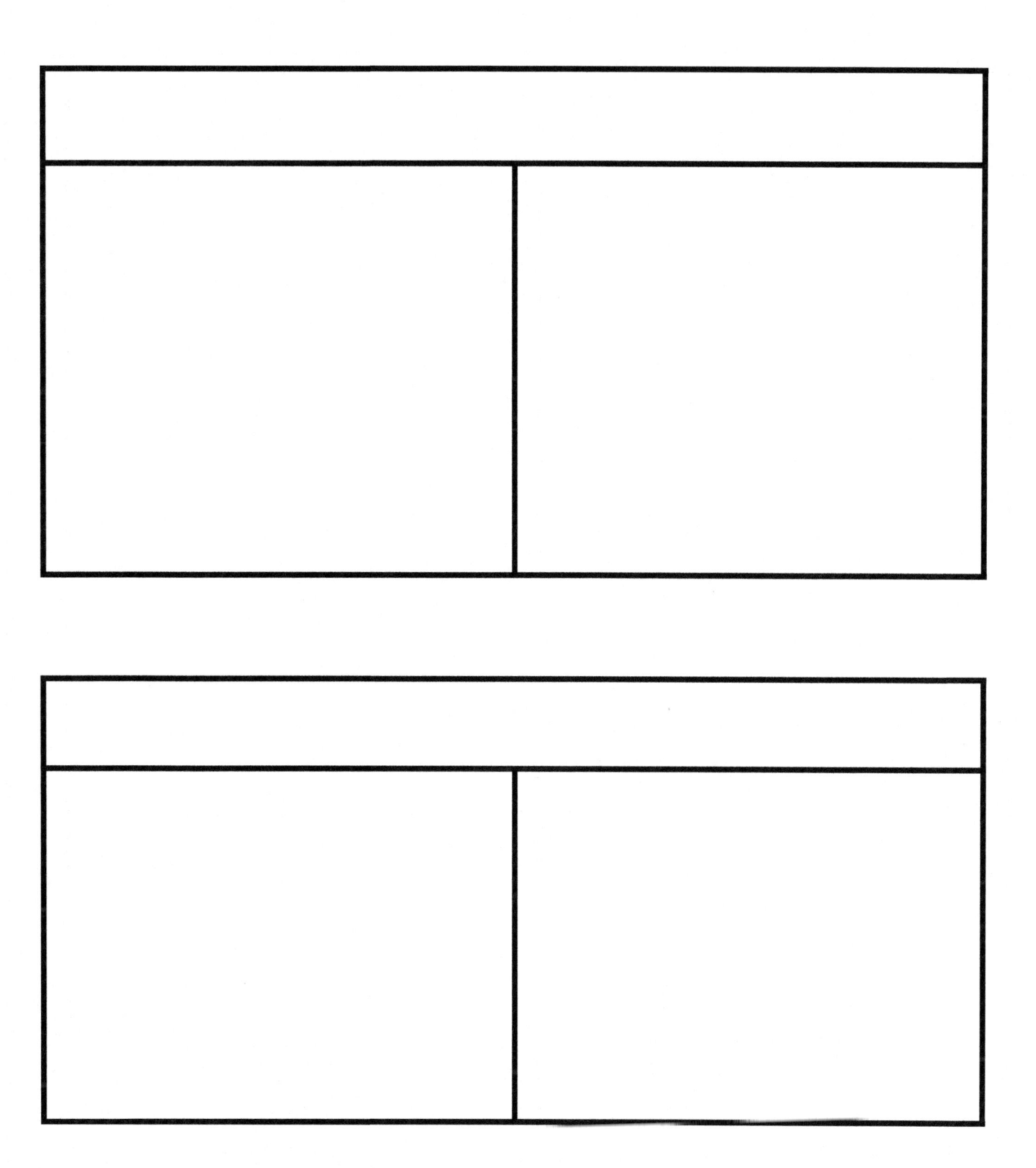

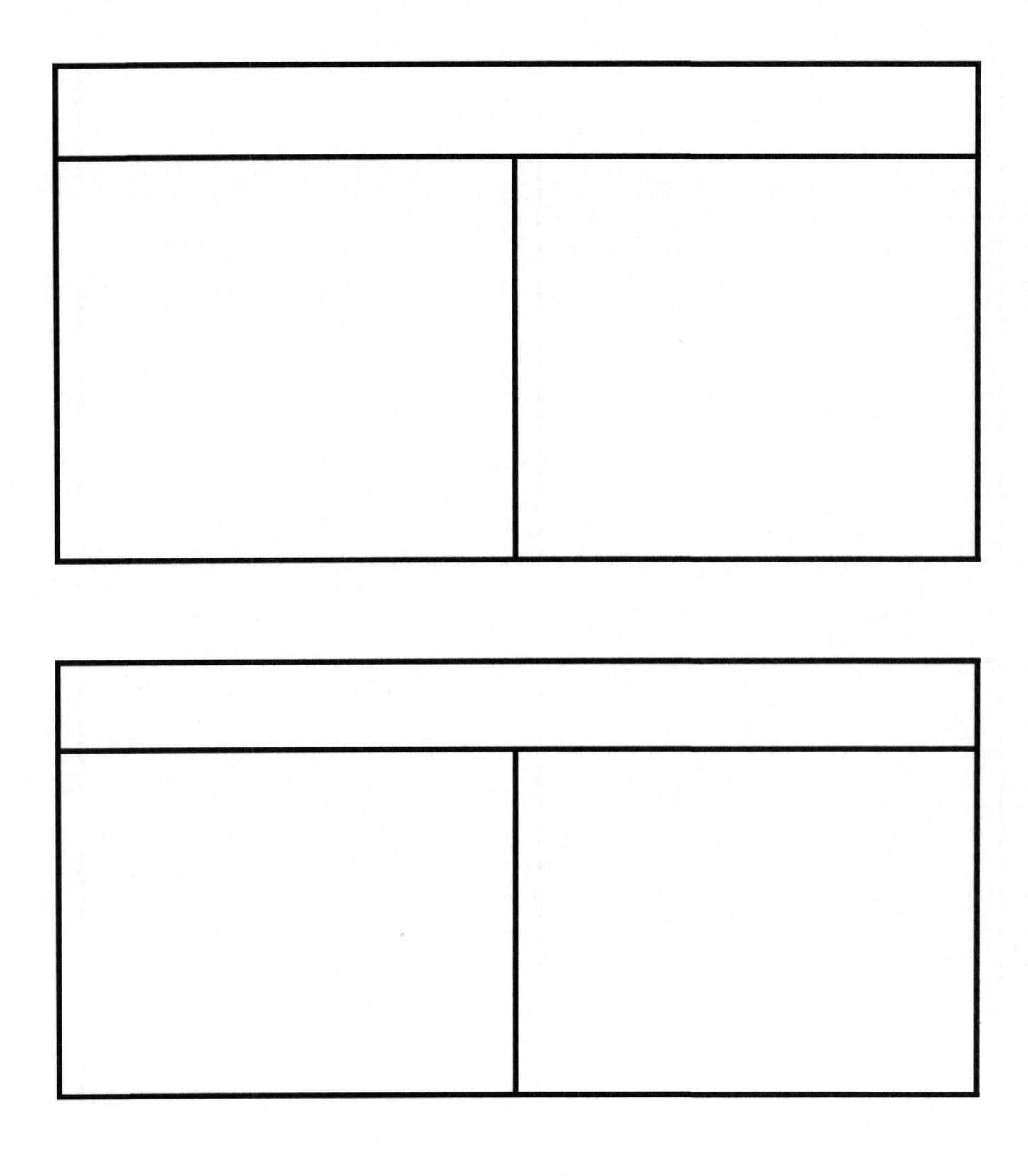

FAVORITE RECIPE JOURNAL

TEMPLATE

RECIPE NAME

INGREDIENTS	INGREDIENTS

COOKING STYLE

PERSONAL TIPS

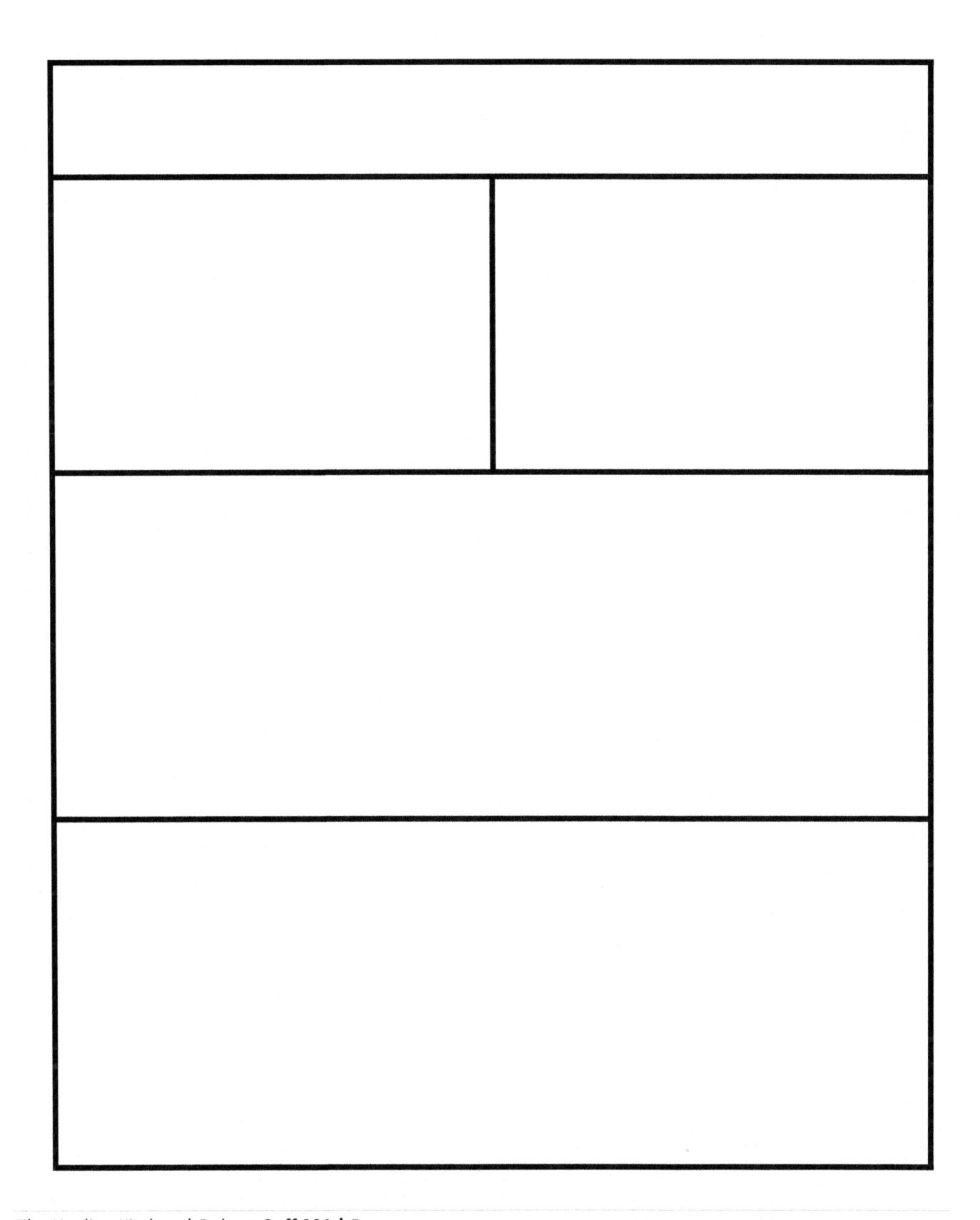

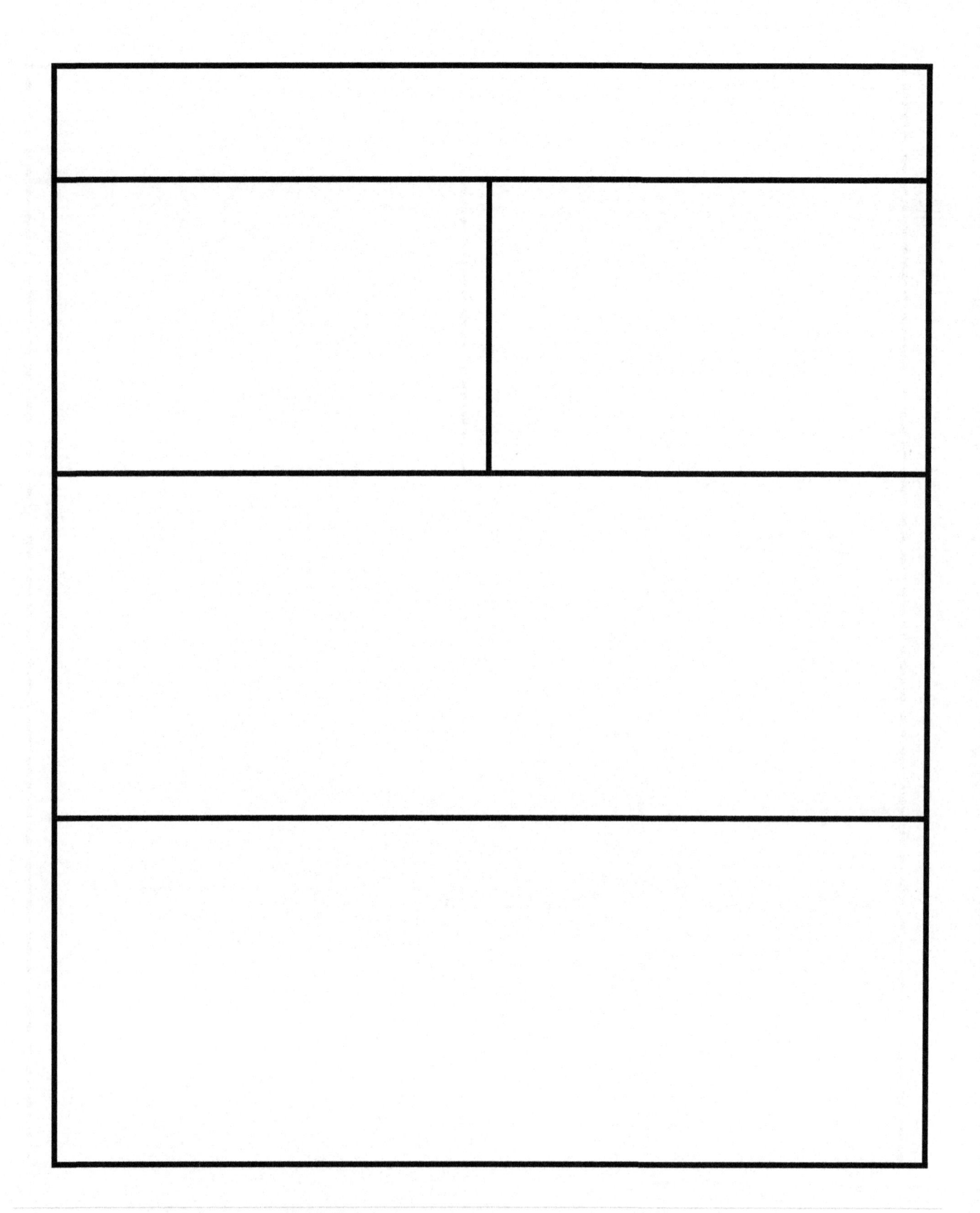

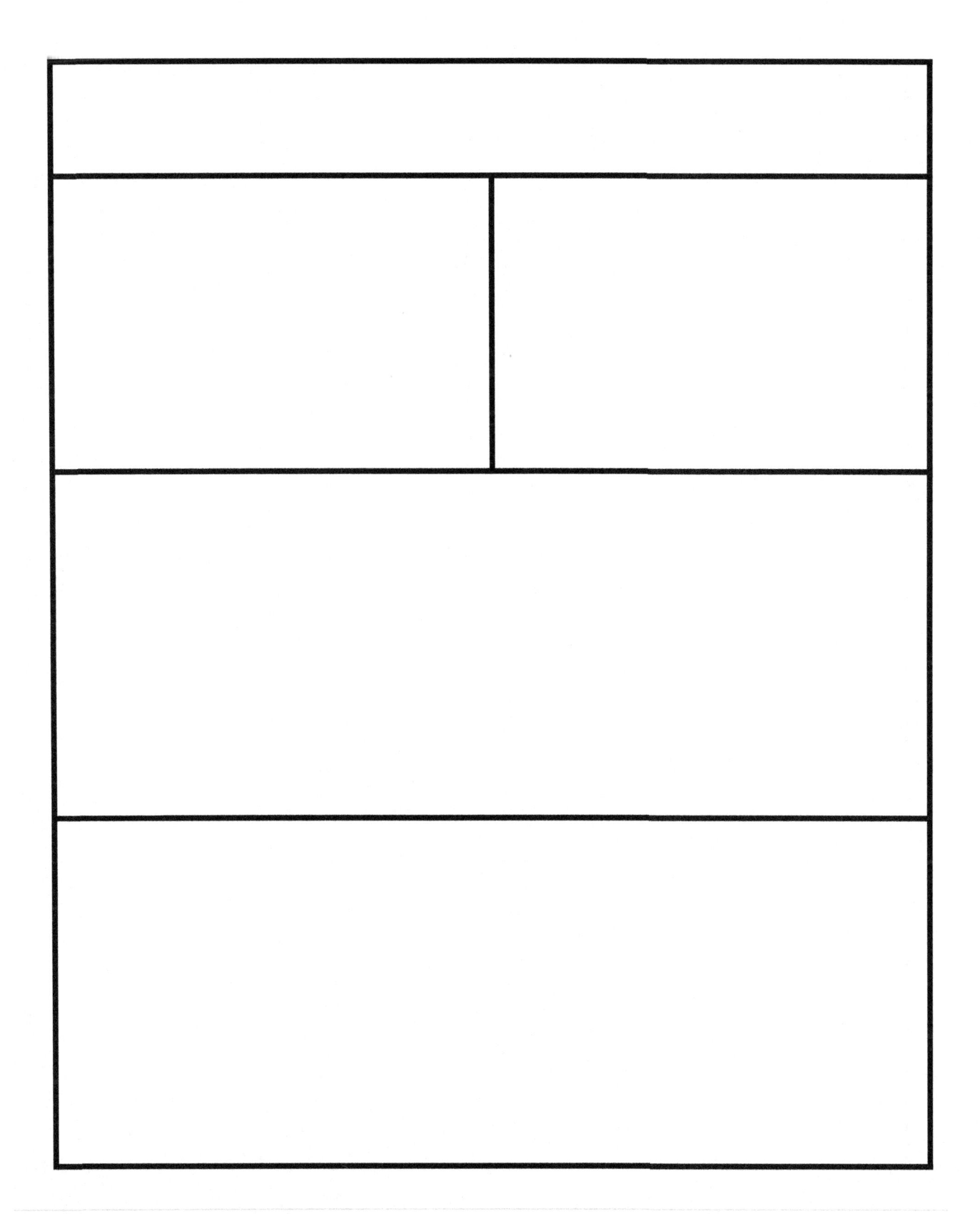

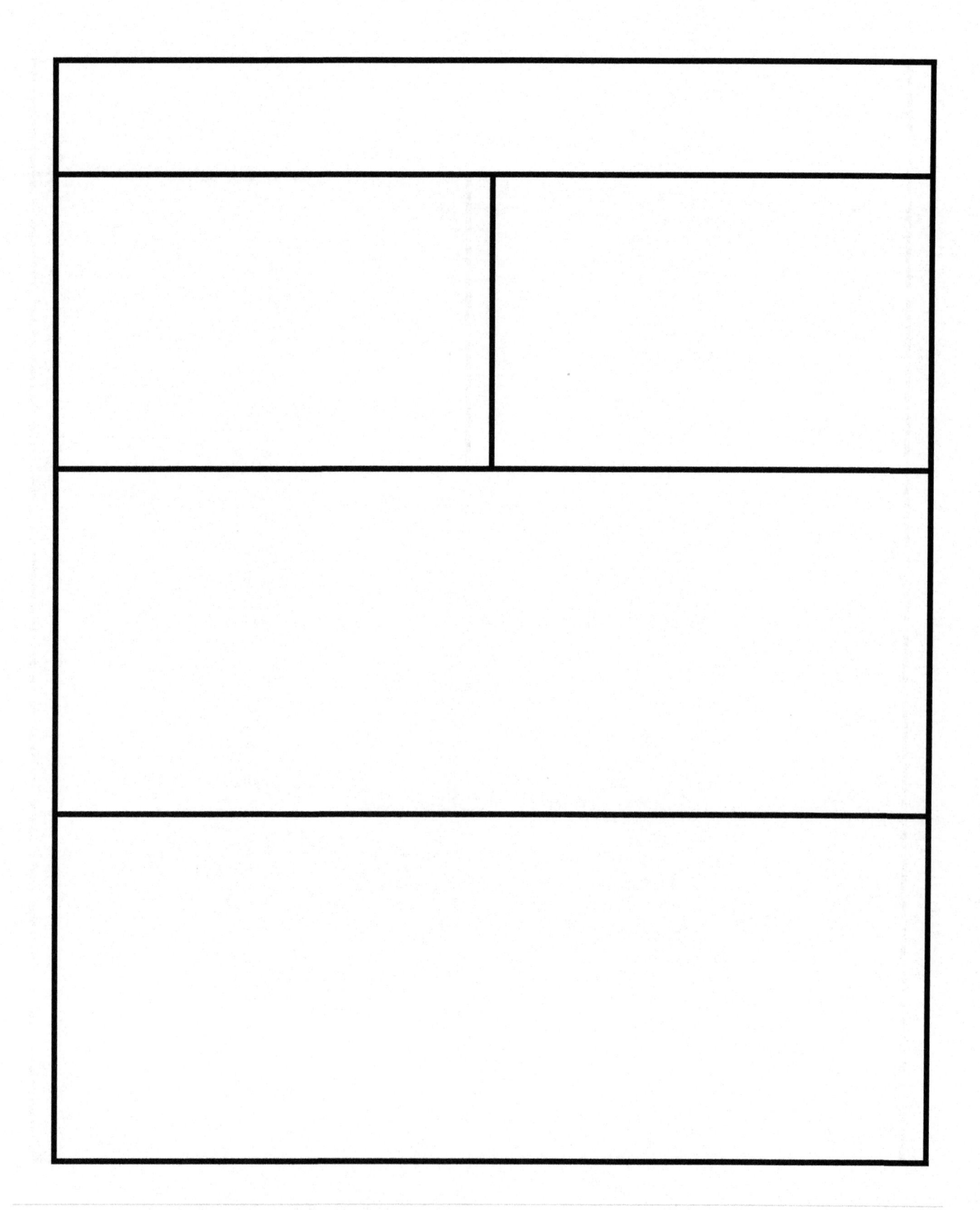

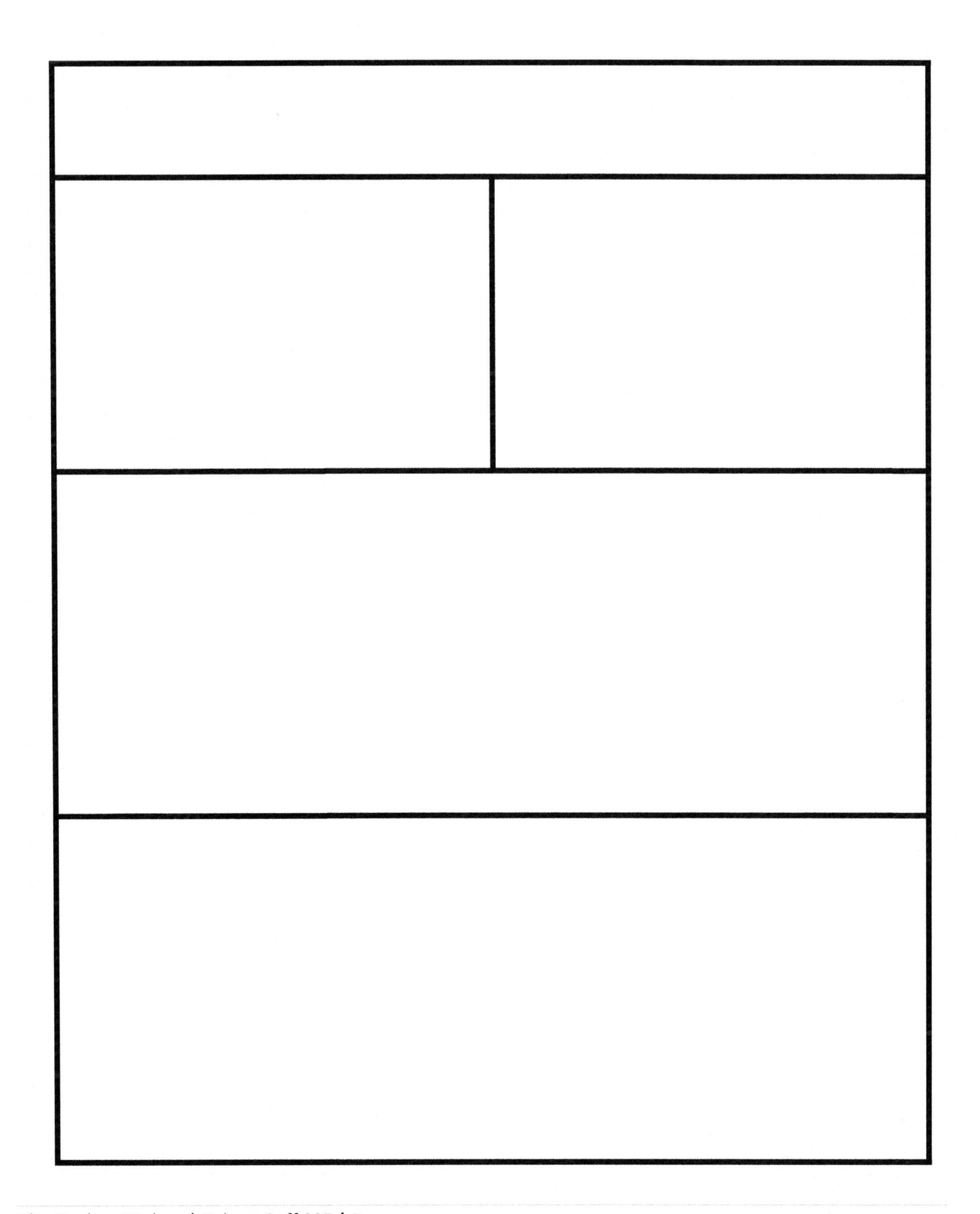

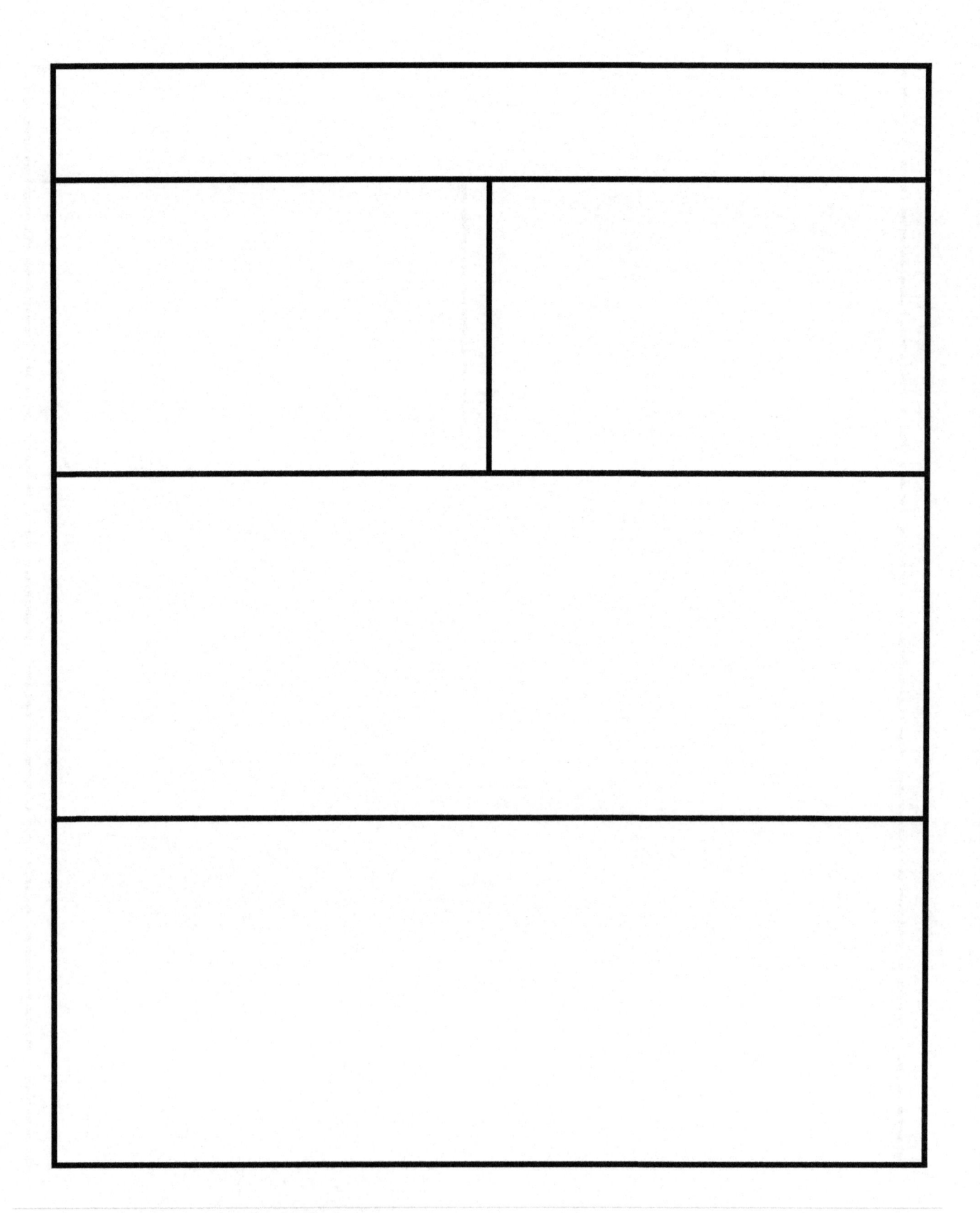

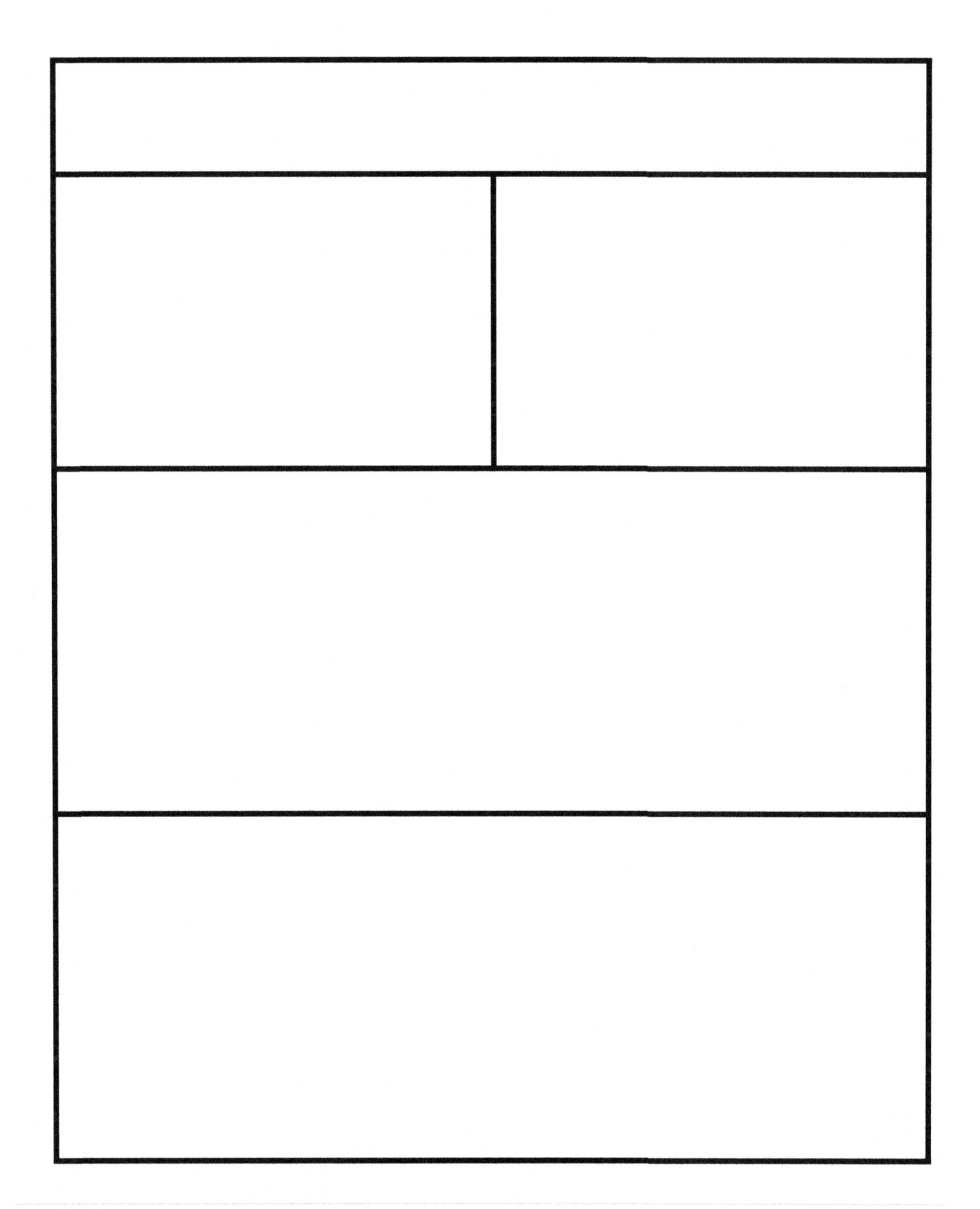

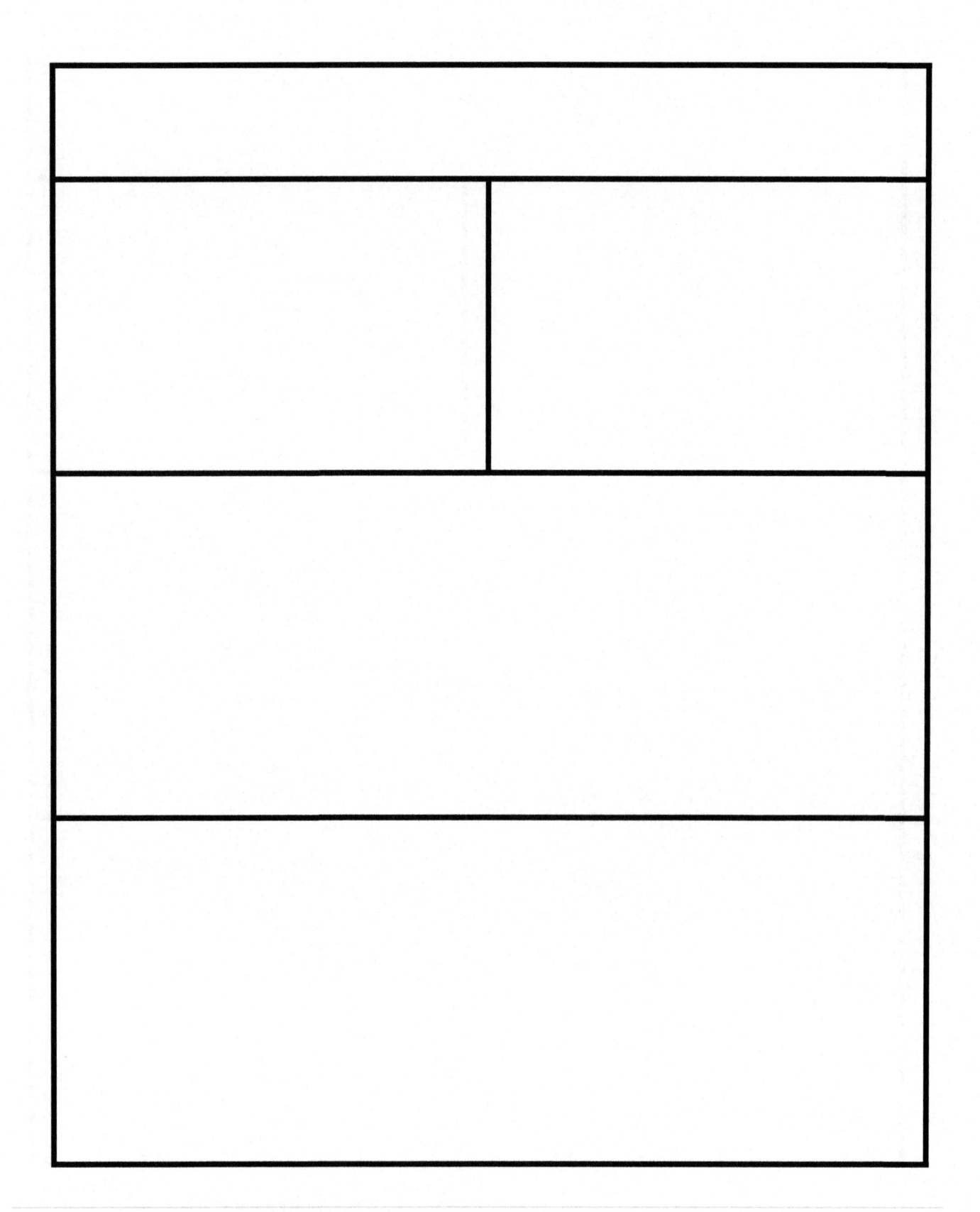

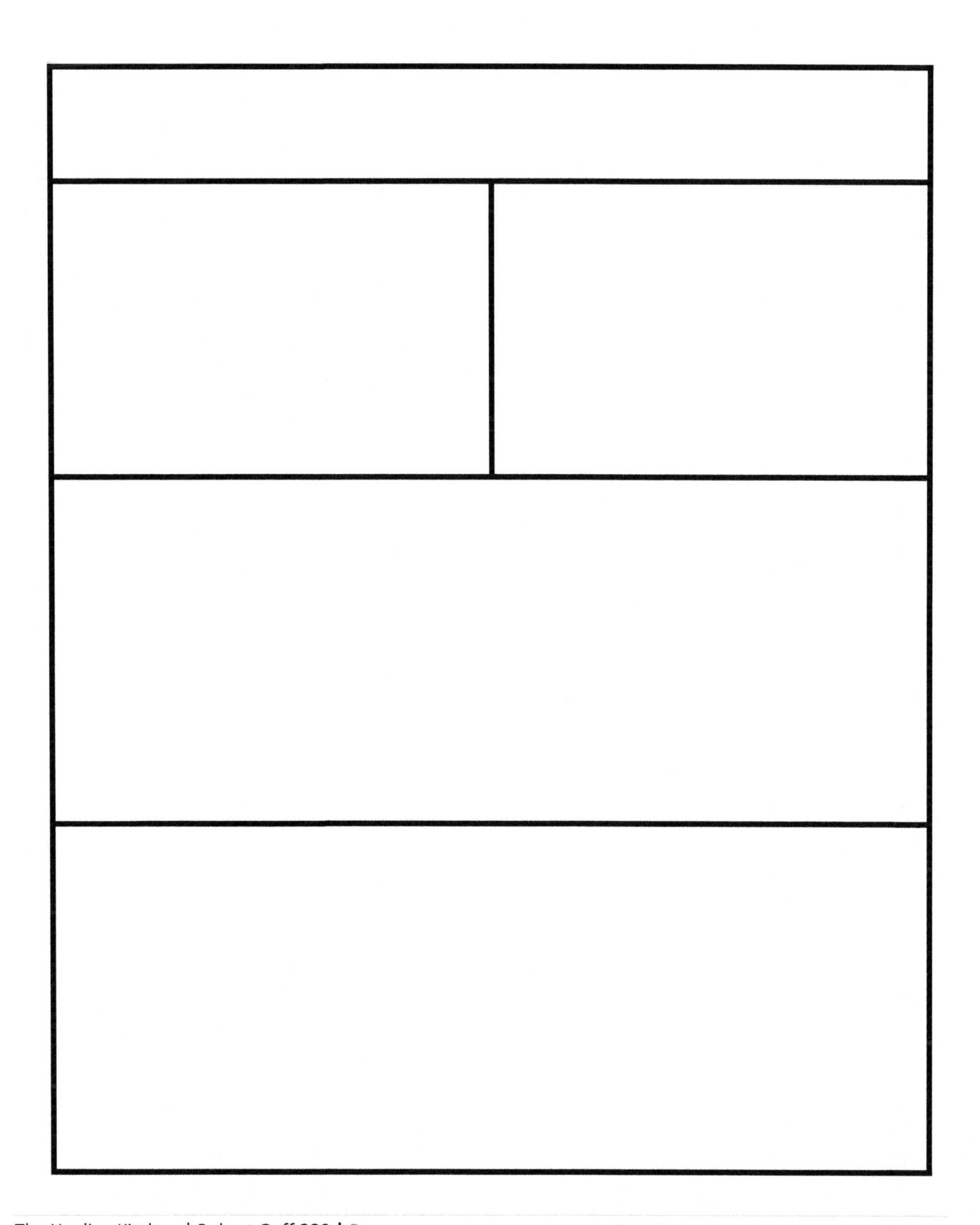

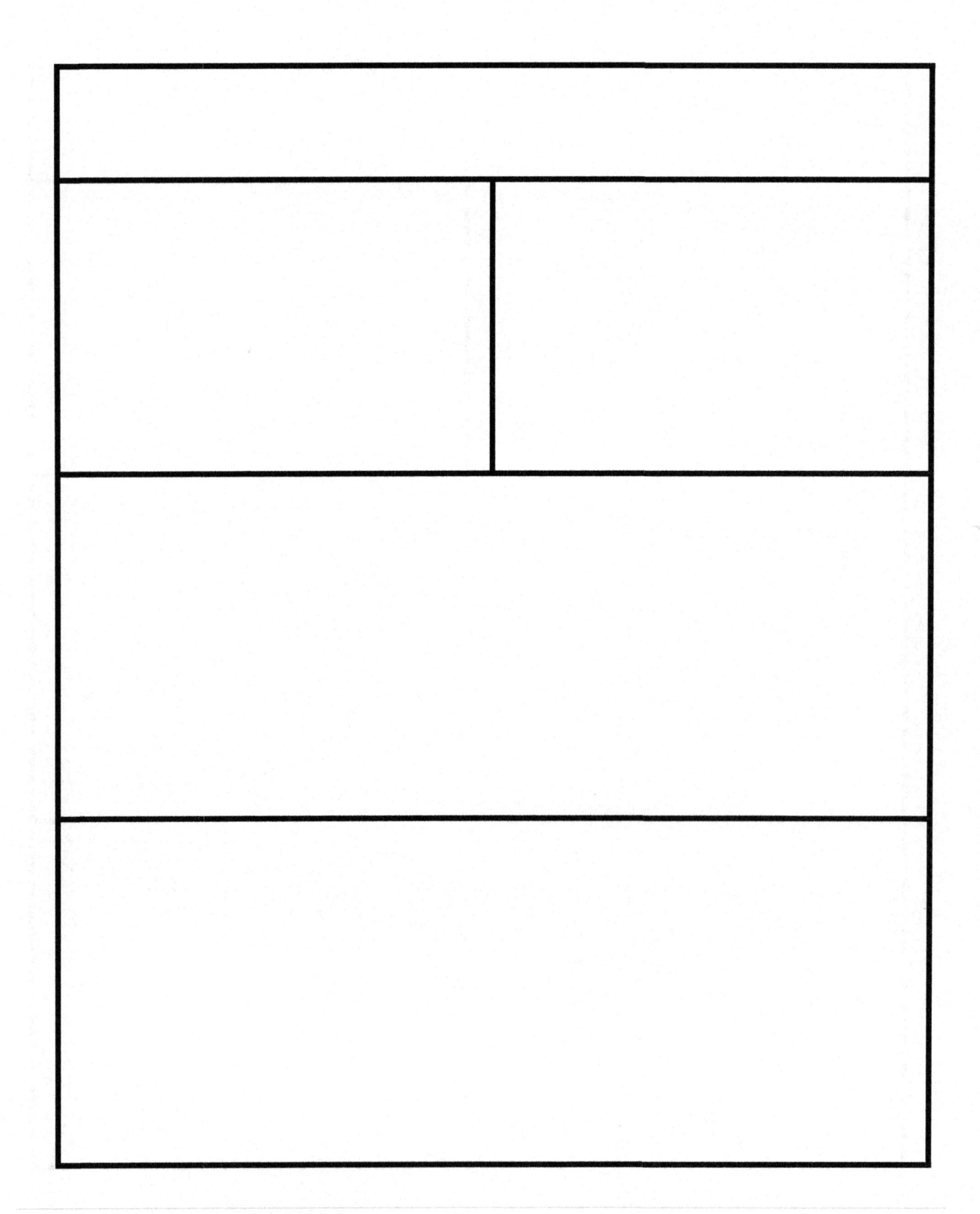

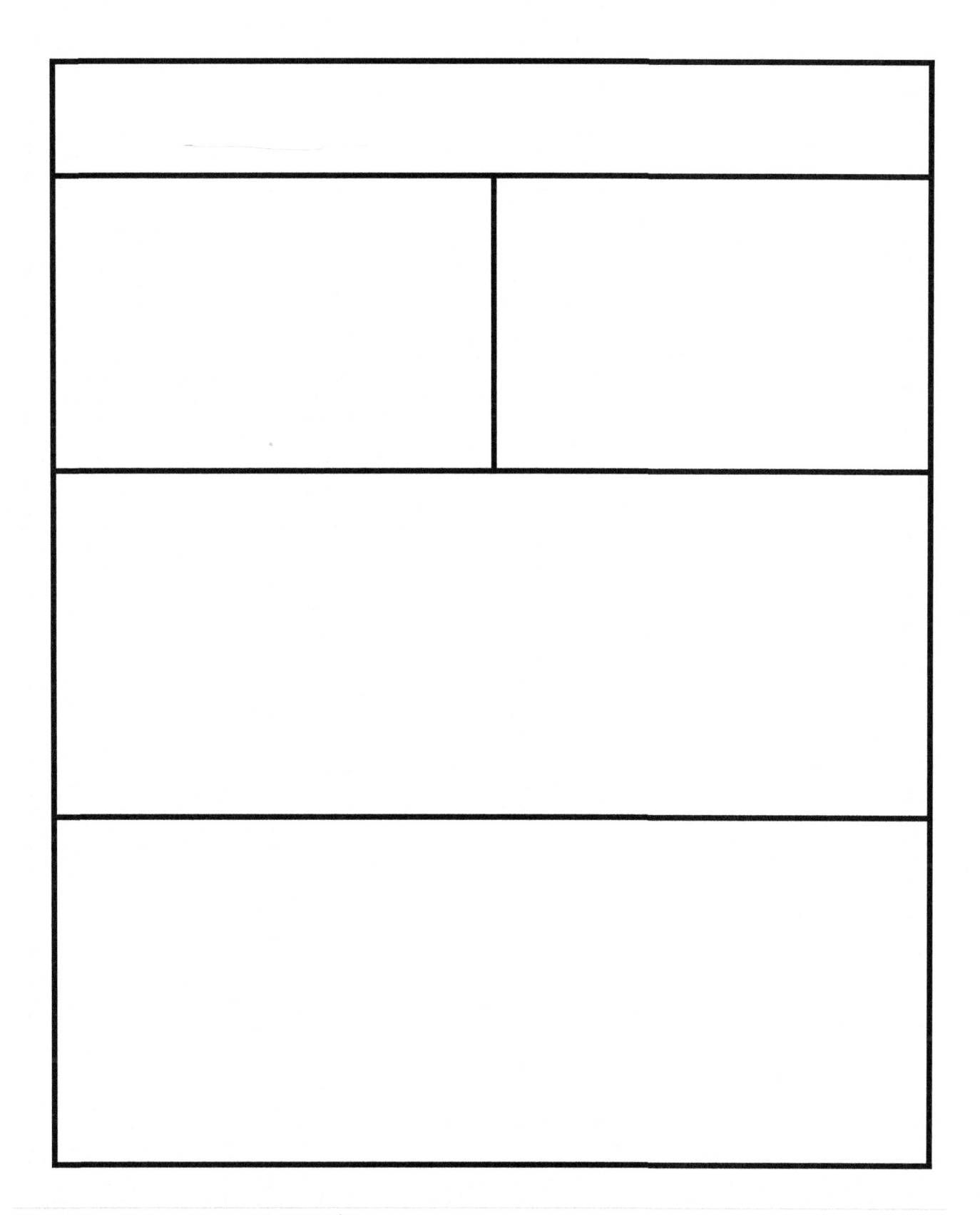

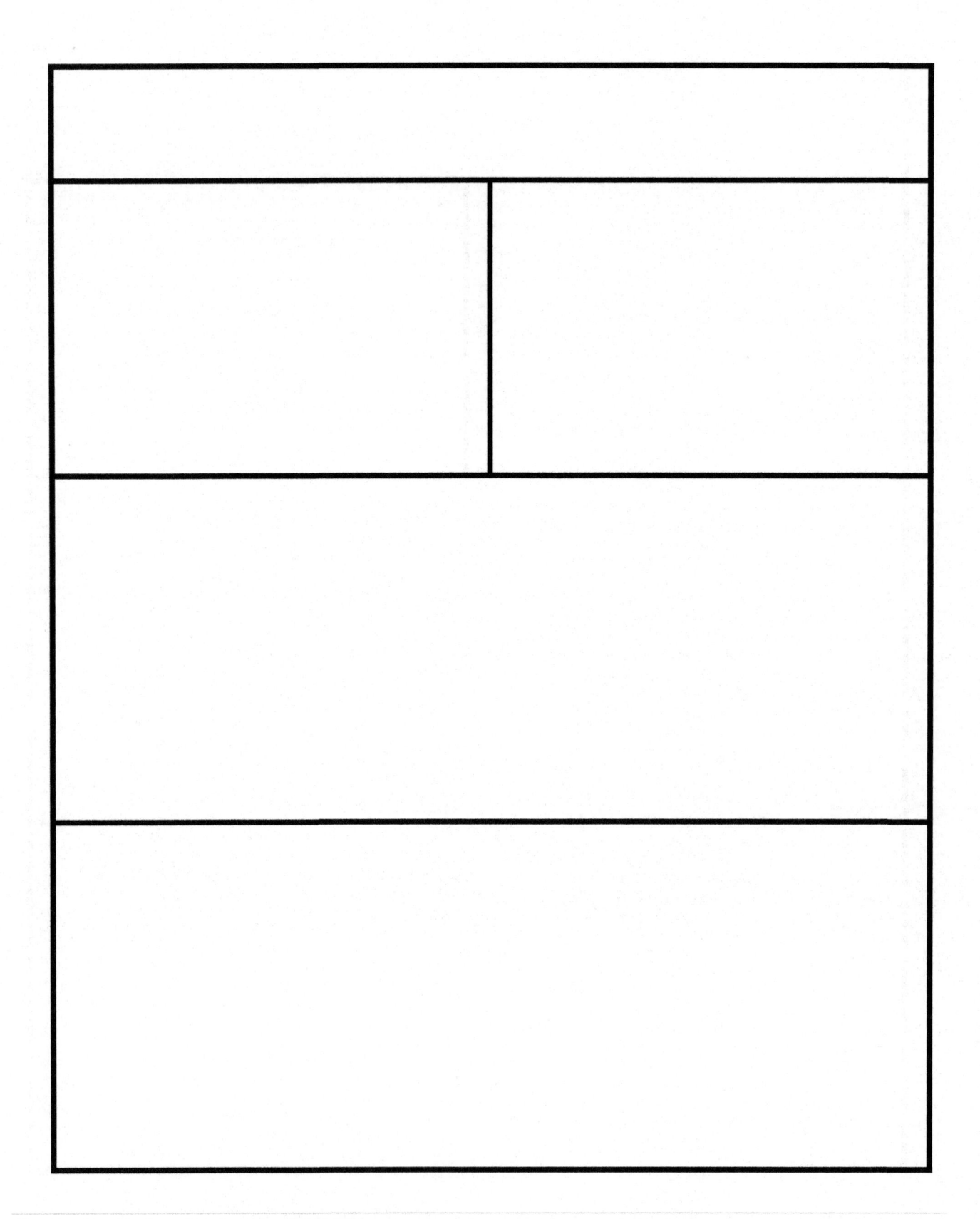

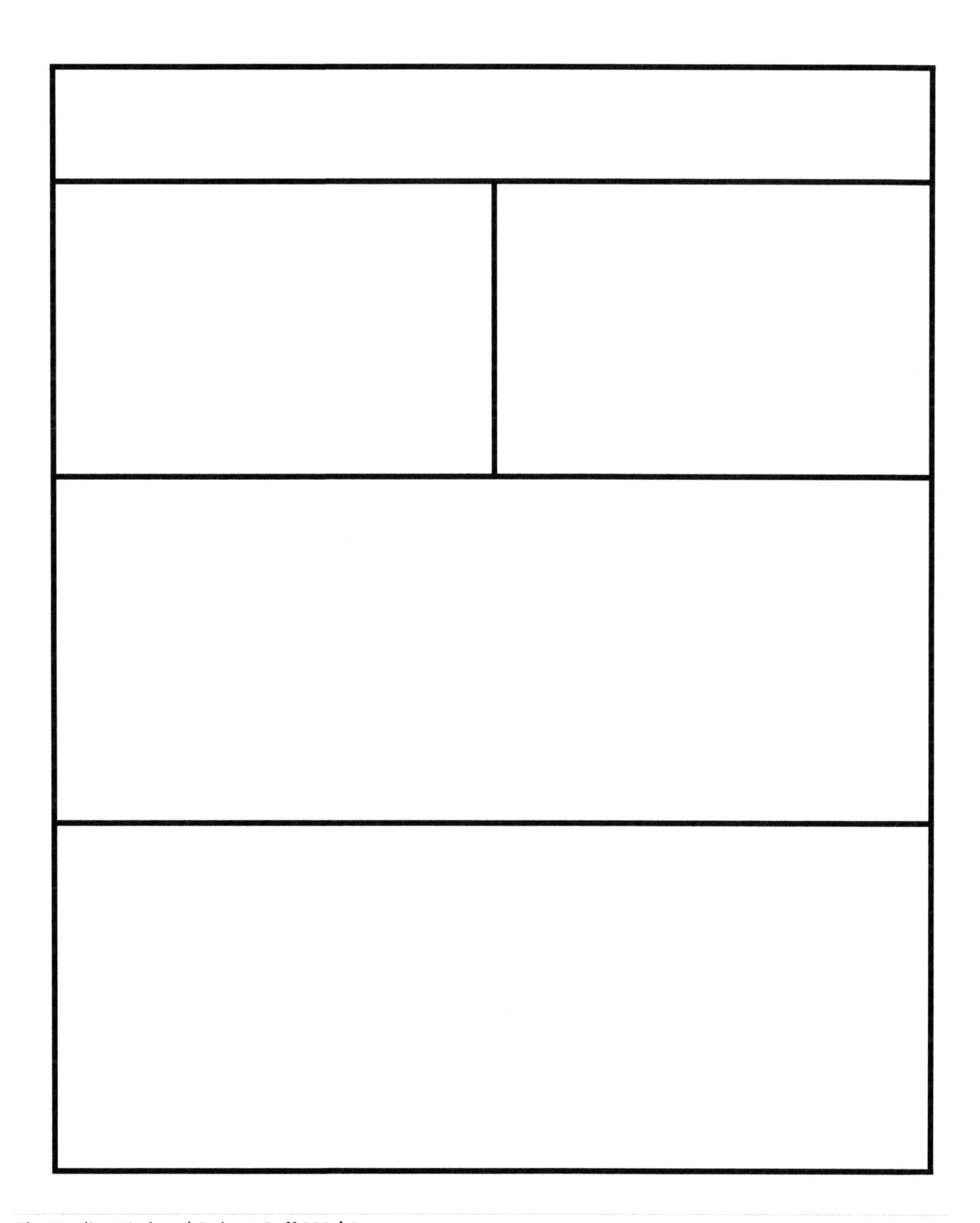

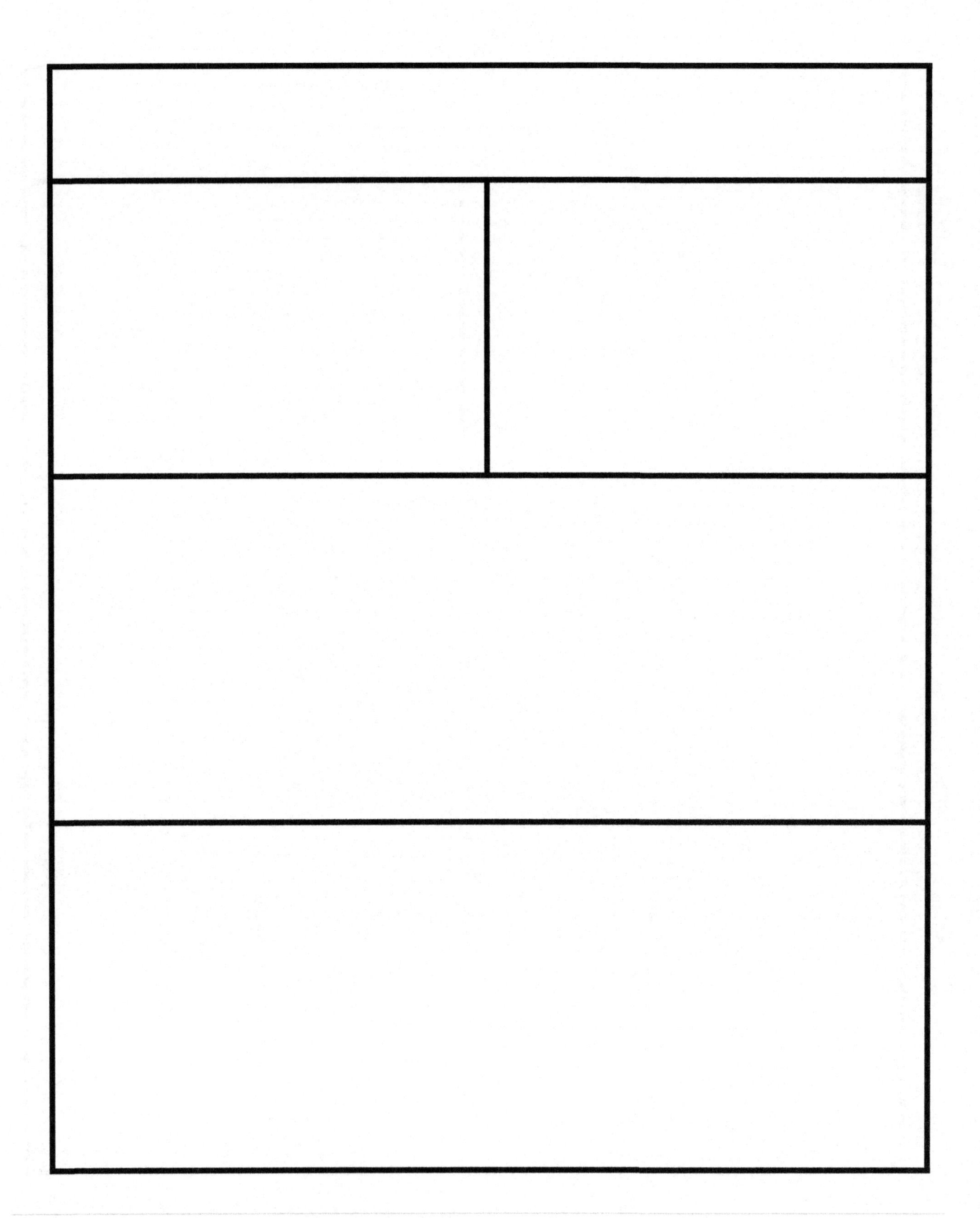

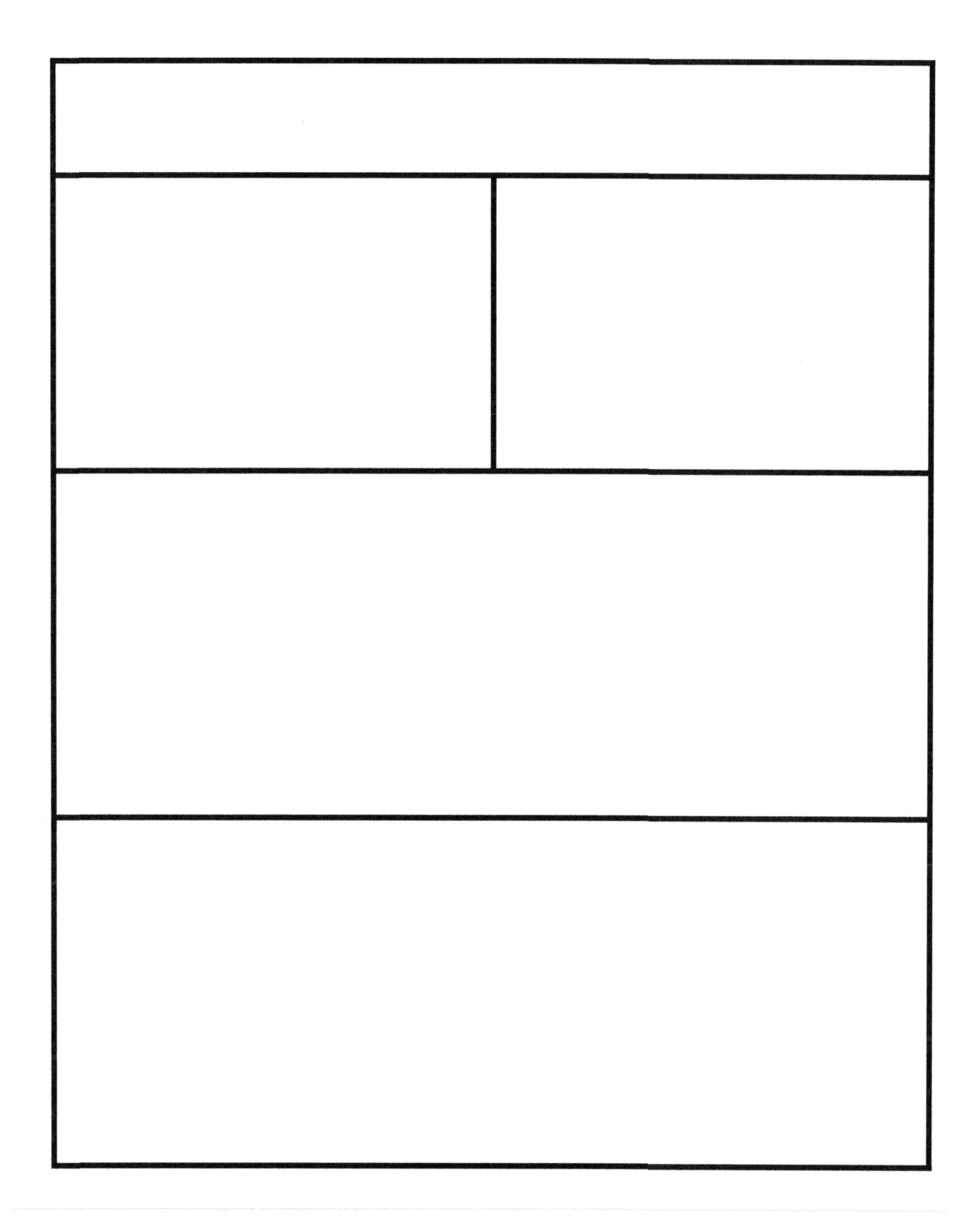

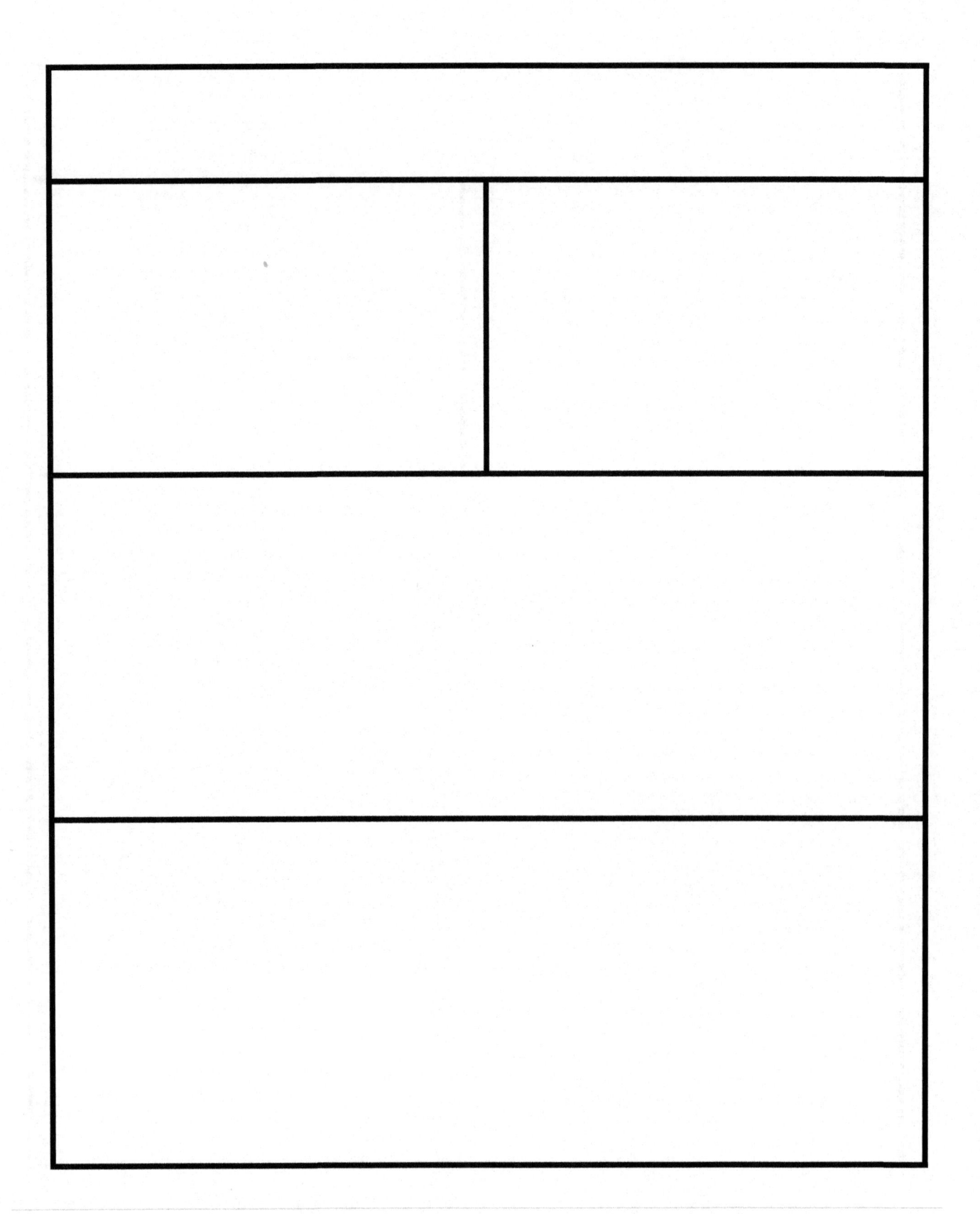

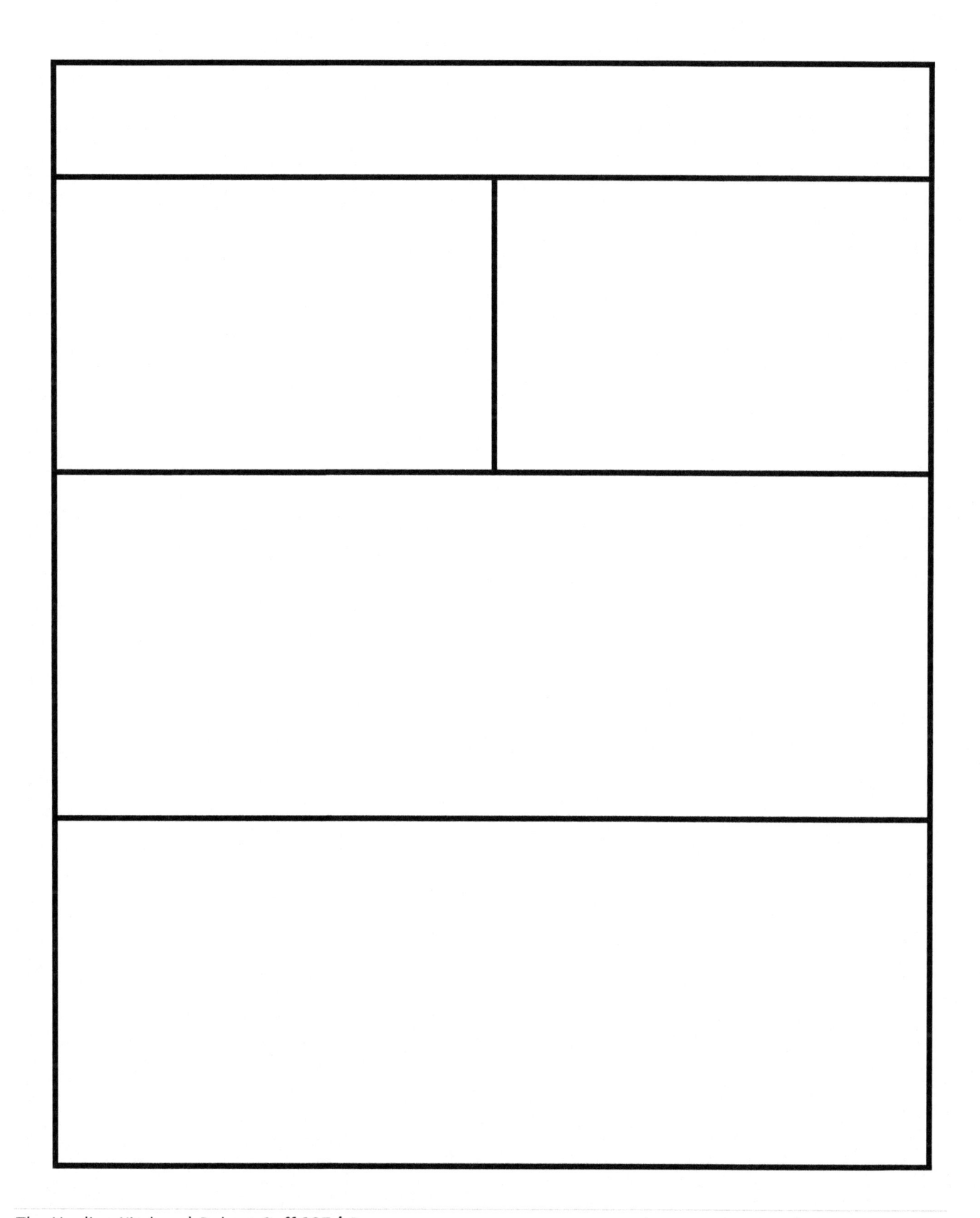

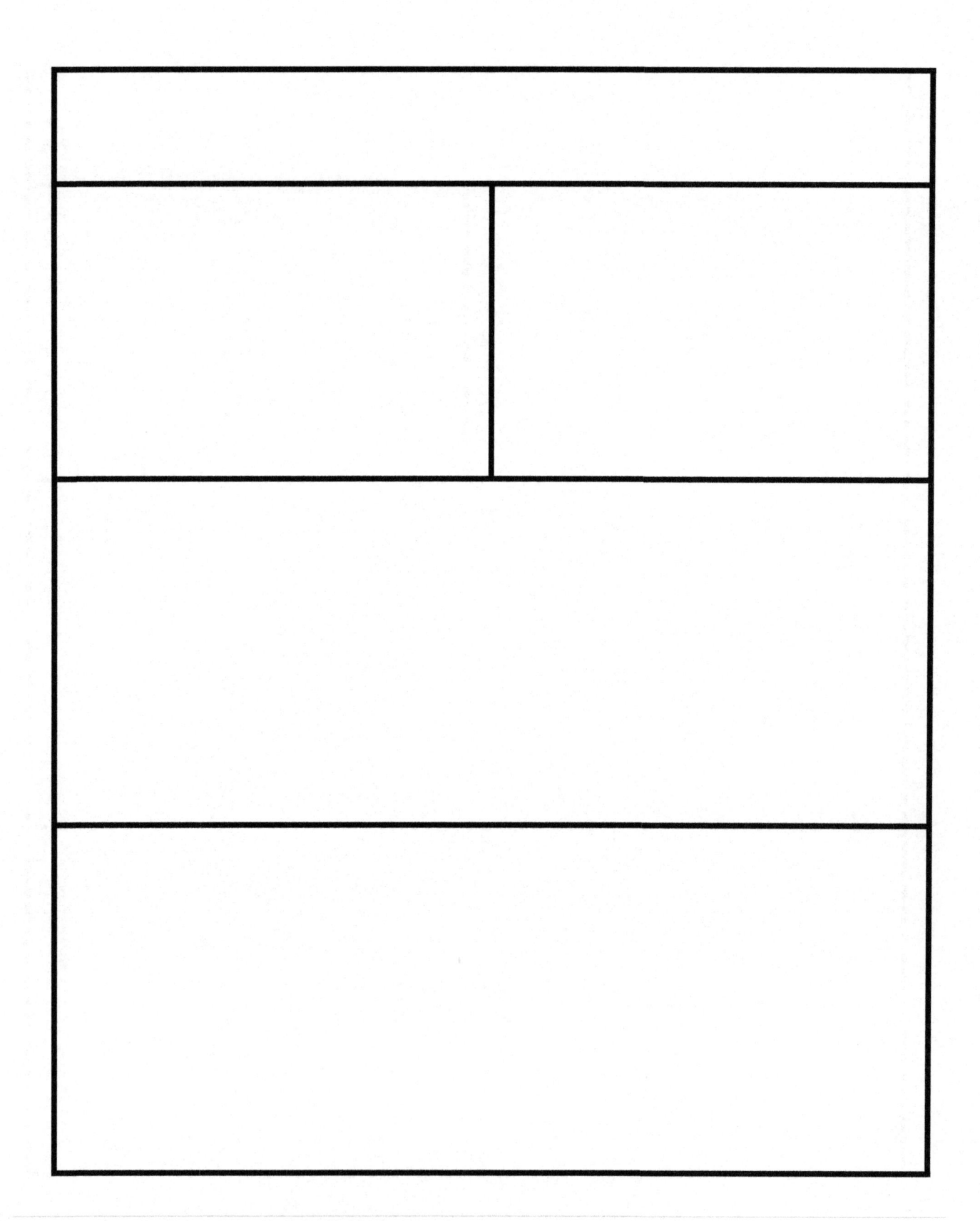

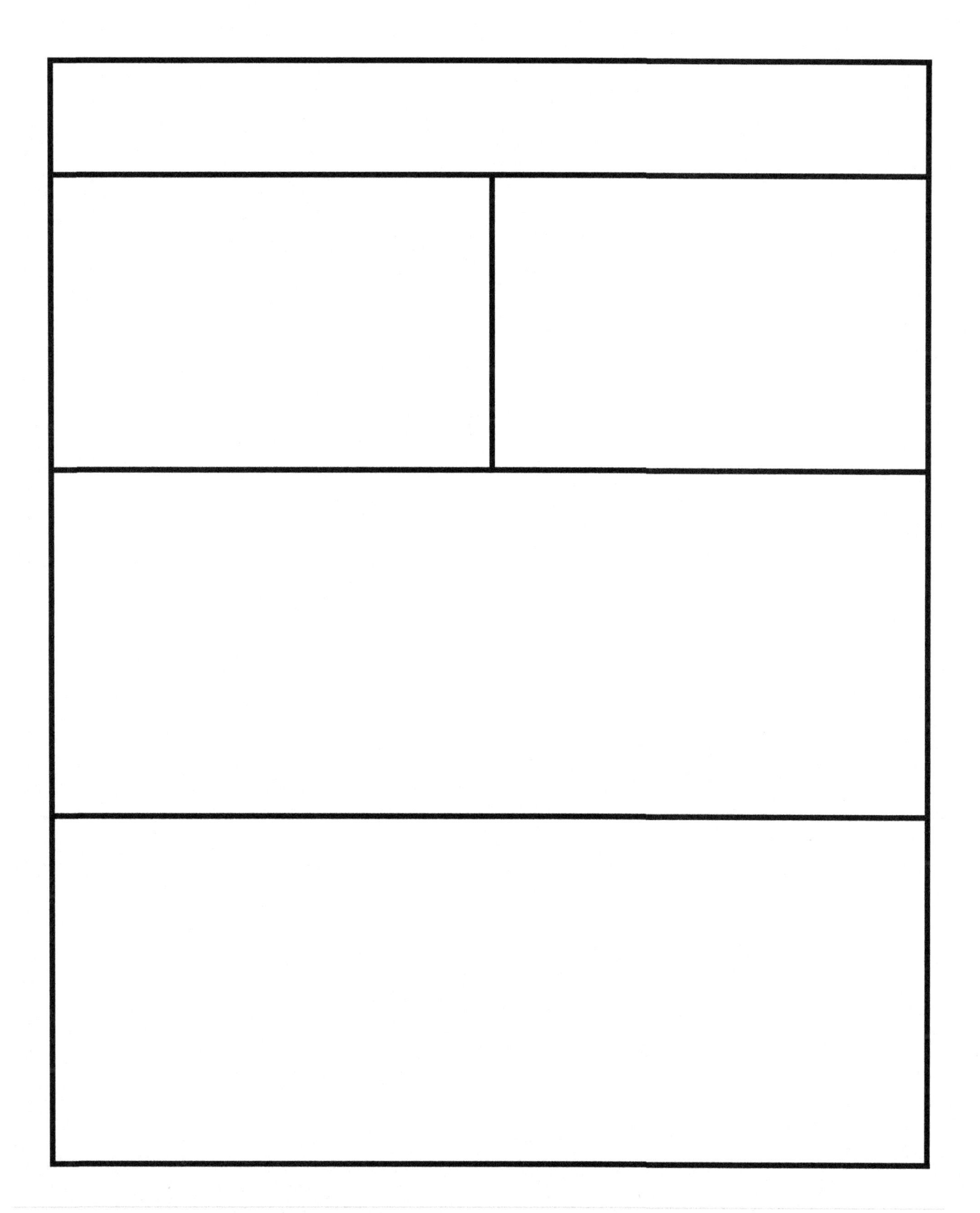

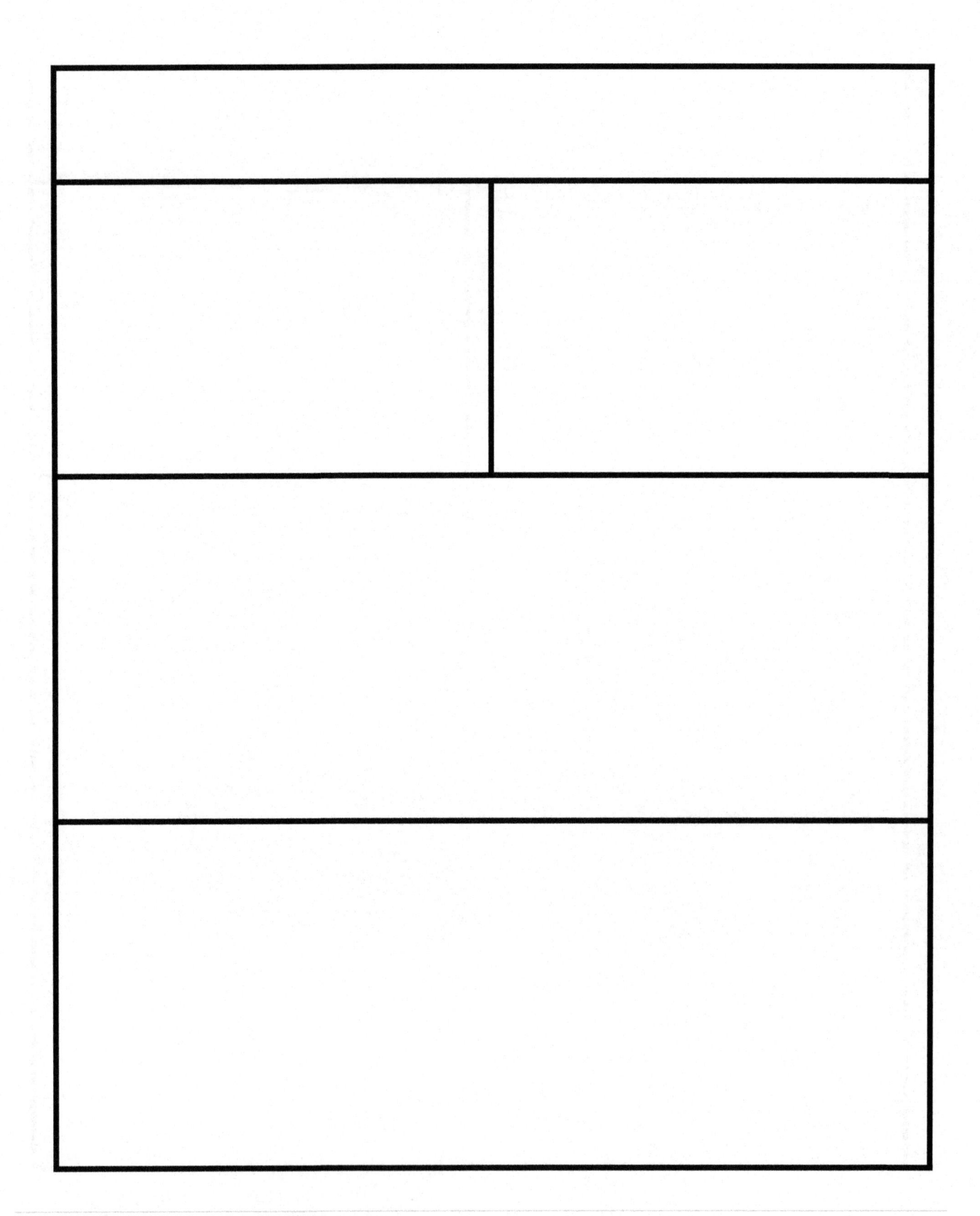

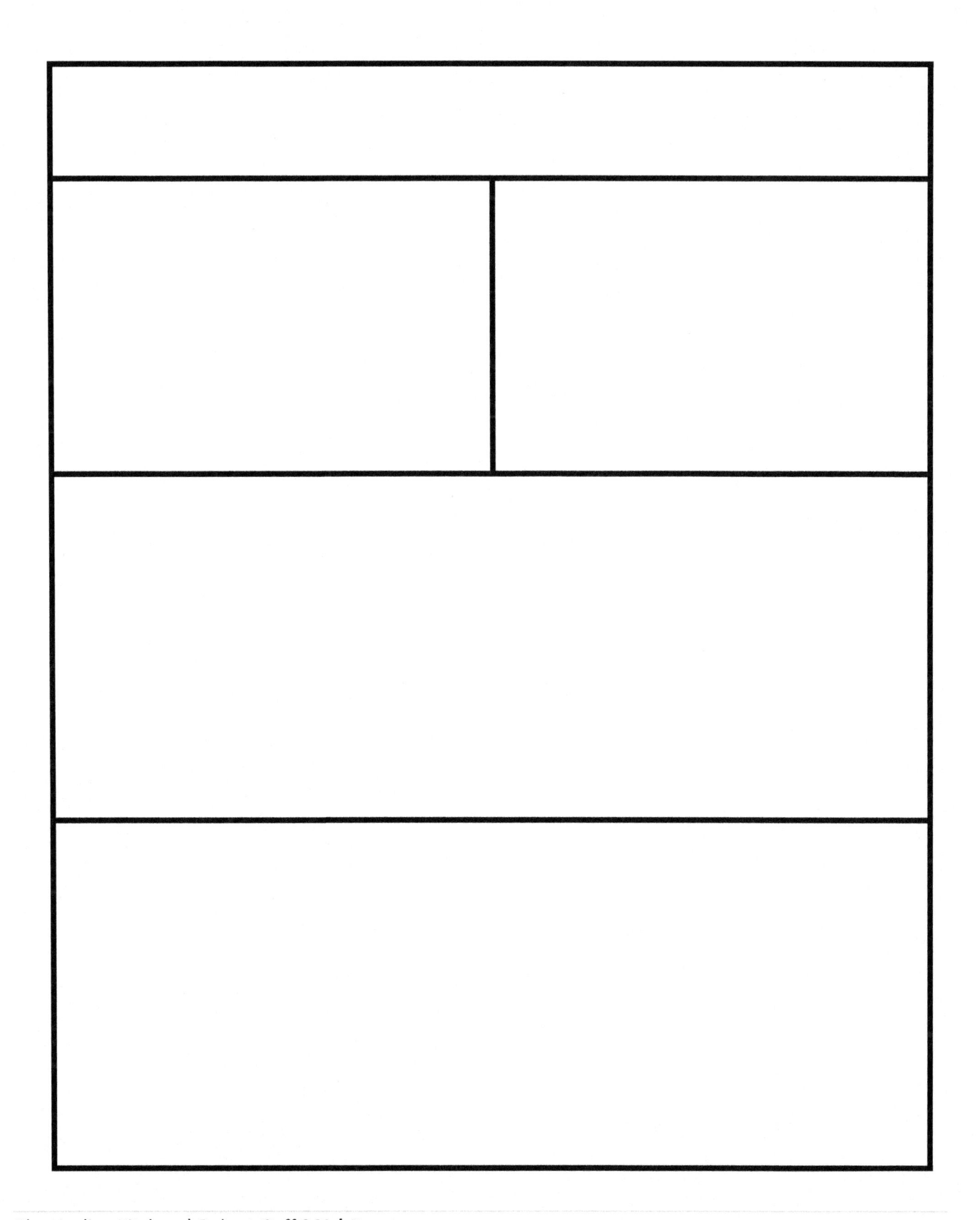

Printed in Great Britain
by Amazon